From John of Apamea to Mark's Gospel

Studies in Biblical Literature

Hemchand Gossai
General Editor

Vol. 160

This book is a volume in a Peter Lang monograph series.
Every volume is peer reviewed and meets
the highest quality standards for content and production.

PETER LANG
New York • Bern • Frankfurt • Berlin
Brussels • Vienna • Oxford • Warsaw

Dempsey Rosales Acosta

From John of Apamea to Mark's Gospel

Two Dialogues with Thomasios: A Hermeneutical Reading of Horáō, Blépō, and Theōréō

PETER LANG
New York • Bern • Frankfurt • Berlin
Brussels • Vienna • Oxford • Warsaw

Library of Congress Cataloging-in-Publication Data

Rosales Acosta, Dempsey.
From John of Apamea to Mark's Gospel: two dialogues with Thomasios:
a hermeneutical reading of Horáo, Blépo, and Theoréo / Dempsey Rosales Acosta.
pages cm. — (Studies in biblical literature; v. 160)
Includes bibliographical references and indexes.
1. John, the Solitary, of Apamea, active 5th century.
2. Bible. Mark—Criticism, interpretation, etc.
3. Vision—Religious aspects—Christianity.
4. Senses and sensation—Religious aspects—Christianity. I. Title.
BR65.Y66R673 230'.14092—dc23 2013046524
ISBN 978-1-4331-2616-1 (hardcover)
ISBN 978-1-4539-1300-0 (e-book)
ISSN 1089-0645

Bibliographic information published by **Die Deutsche Nationalbibliothek**.
Die Deutsche Nationalbibliothek lists this publication in the "Deutsche Nationalbibliografie"; detailed bibliographic data are available on the Internet at http://dnb.d-nb.de/.

The paper in this book meets the guidelines for permanence and durability of the Committee on Production Guidelines for Book Longevity of the Council of Library Resources.

29 Broadway, 18th floor, New York, NY 10006
www.peterlang.com

Printed in Germany

"Imagine that there is nothing else in front of your eyes—as though you were not among humankind—because you are seeing nothing else but God, for God is the entire reason for your way of life"

John the Solitary, *Letter to Hesychius*, 17

In honor of Roberto Lückert, Lisa and Maria Betita

Table of Contents

Editor's Preface

More than ever the horizons in biblical literature are being expanded beyond that which is immediately imagined; important new methodological, theological, and hermeneutical directions are being explored, often resulting in significant contributions to the world of biblical scholarship. It is an exciting time for the academy as engagement in biblical studies continues to be heightened.

This series seeks to make available to scholars and institutions, scholarship of a high order, and which will make a significant contribution to the ongoing biblical discourse. This series includes established and innovative directions, covering general and particular areas in biblical study. For every volume considered for this series, we explore the question as to whether the study will push the horizons of biblical scholarship. The answer must be yes for inclusion.

In this volume Dempsey Rosales Acosta explores the works of the little known and studied work of John of Apamea. Using the methodological approach that is termed "spiritual exegesis," the author explores the use of horáō, blépō, and theōréo in the Gospel of Mark, seeking to understand the notion of visual perception. It is Acosta's contention that the theological conceptions of John of Apamea serve as the hermeneutical lenses through which the Gospel of Mark might be most faithfully interpreted and understood. One of interests in this study will be the potential scholarly impact on Markan scholarship as the variety of methodologies and lenses continue to expand. I believe that this study will be of benefit to both the academy and the Church.

The horizon has been expanded.

Hemchand Gossai

Series Editor

Acknowledgements

Gratitude is a virtue that must be cultivated in every field of life, and any moment can be used as the appropriate time to practice it. For this reason it is necessary to acknowledge my gratitude to several people who have been valuable instruments in the elaboration and finalization of this research.

First of all I want to express my gratefulness to Archbishop Roberto Lückert León who has been a decisive instrument in my dedication to the study of Theology and biblical exegesis. I am especially grateful to Dr. Mario Paredes, President of the American Bible Society's Presidential Liaison for Roman Catholic Ministries and chairman of the Board of the Catholic Association of Latino Leaders (CALL), who, since 2010, has provided me with opportunities to present my work to different specialized audiences who in turn have challenged me to refine and develop the theological themes that have acquired their final form in this present book. It was during that period of time when the fundamental elements of this book began to be formulated. To Dr. Hemchand Gossai who has made possible the publication of this work with his suggestions and comments.

I thank my former professor Dr. Elena Bosetti who was the first university lecturer that opened my eyes to Mark's Gospel through her teaching and works when I used to be her student at the Pontifical Gregorian University. I am also grateful to my assistant, Ms. Esther Hudson, whose enthusiasm for the project and helpful comments have helped to make this text more understandable in this English version.

Abbreviations

ABR	Australian Biblical Review
ACCS	Ancient Christian Commentary on Scripture
AEMA	Archivum Eurasiae Medii Aevi
AnBib	Analecta Biblica. Editrice Pontificio Istituto Biblico. Roma
AncB	The Anchor Bible Series. Garden City, NY: Doubleday
BAC	Biblioteca de Autores Cristianos. Madrid
BAGD	Bauer, Walter, Arndt, William, and Gingrich, Wilburg. A Greek-English Lexicon of the New Testament and Other Early Christian Literature, 2nd Edition. Chicago – London: Chicago University Press, 1979
Bib	Biblica. Pontificio Istituto Biblico. Roma
BJRL	Bulletin of the John Rylands (University) Library
Blass-Debrunner	Grammatica del Greco del Nuevo Testamento. Edited by Friederich Rehkopf. Brescia: Paideia, 1997
BSOAS	Bulletin of the School of Oriental and African Studies
CCC	Catechism of the Catholic Church
C. Cels.	Contra Celsum. Origen
CCSL	Corpus Christianorum Series Latina
CSCO	Corpus Scriptorum Christianorum Orientalium
CUA	Catholic University of America
DENT	Diccionario Exegético del Nuevo Testamento (eds. Balz, H. – Schneider, G.)
DSAM	Dictionnaire de Spiritualité Ascétique et Mystique (Ascetic Spirituality and Mysticism Dictionary)
EWNT	Exegetisches Wörterbuch zum Neuen Testament
FC	Fathers of the Church: A New Translation, 86 vols.Catholic University of America Press, 1947-

JAAS	Journal of Assyrian Academic Studies
JAOS	Journal of the American Oriental Society
JECS	Journal of Eastern Christian Studies
JETS	Journal of the Evangelical Theological Society
LXX	Septuagint
NIGTC	The New International Greek Testament Commentary
NJBC	The New Jerome Biblical Commentary, edited by Raymond Brown, Joseph Fitzmyer, and Roland Murphy. Englewood Cliffs, NJ: Prentice-Hall/ Simon & Schuster, 1988.
NT	New Testament
NPNF	A Select Library of the Nicene and Post-Nicene Fathers of the Christian Church, edited by P. Schaff et al. Reprint, Peabody, Mass.: Hendrickson, 1994
OCA	Orientalia Christiana Analecta
OCP	Orientalia Christiana Periodica
OLP	Orientalia Lovaniensia Periodica
OT	Old Testament
PO	Parole de l'Orient
PG	Patrologia Graeca: Patrologiae Cursus Completus, Series Graeca, edited by Jacques Paul Migne, 1857-1866
PL	Patrologia Latina: Patrologiae Cursus Completus, Series Latina, edited by Jacques Paul Migne, 1857-1866
PLS	Patrologiae Latinae Suplementum
PTS	Patristiche Texte und Studien
RAM	Revue d'Ascétique et de Mystique
RScR	Recherches des Sciences Religieuse
ROC	Revue de l'Orient Chrétien
SC	Sources Chrétiennes

SNTW	Studies of the New Testament and its World
TDNT	Kittel, G. and Friedrich, G., eds. Theological Dictionary of the New Testament , translated by G. Bromiley. Grand Rapids, MI: William B. Eerdmans, 1985
THNT	Theologischer Handkommentar zum Neuen Testament
ThS	Theological Studies
ThZ	Theologische Zeitschrift, Basel
UTB	Urban Taschenbuch
VGNT	Vocabulary of the Greek New Testament
VT	Vetus Testamentum, Leiden
ZDMG	Zeitschrift der Deutschen Morgenländischen Gesellschaft

Introduction

The present work elucidates upon the relation between two theological fields that are connected through their very nature, for one builds its theological conclusions upon the other. The first field of research is related to Patristic theology, particularly focused on the Eastern writings of an enigmatic monk, who can be identified by the name John of Apamea. The second theological field resides in the discipline of Biblical Theology. For the sake of clarity and precision, the present investigation is delimited to the analysis of selected pericopes of the Gospel of Mark where the verbs of visual perception, i.e., Horáō, Blépō, and Theōréō, are found and these become the semantic objects of this study.

The research presents these two fields complementing each other in a logical line of exposition in which the theological conceptions of the Syrian Monk serve as the hermeneutical key for reading the Gospel of Mark. The results of the investigation come from the approach known as "spiritual exegesis," which has been applied to the narrative of this Gospel of Mark. Such a biblical approach was very common during the Patristic era, being one of the most valid and fruitful ways of understanding, living, and studying the Scripture. It is common to think in our modern times that this form of exegesis is invalid because it lacks scientific and objective grounds and results. Modern exegetical methods can be very useful in helping to discover the process of formation of the text, its historical context, its life setting or Sitz im Leben, its authorship, etc., but many times these methodological readings lose sight of the true intent of the final written texts.

The purpose of the Scripture is to transmit a message of faith. The revelation or experience of God manifested in the written text becomes a source of spirituality that encourages the reader to grow closer to the mystery manifested in its lines. In ancient times, the fathers kept this primary intention as a permanent idea in their biblical elucidations. Their reading of the Scripture was serious and objective since they paid close attention to the text itself, which hides multiple meanings that God uses to communicate to each reader. Thus, their study does not deny the importance of the literal analysis of the sacred text; on the contrary, it presupposes it as a platform upon which the spiritual reflection takes place. This theological point of view to the reading of the Scripture is typical of John of Apamea.

A pattern that has become standard in many books on Christian history in the United States, Western Europe, and Latin America is the presentation of the Christian tradition under two basic historical branches: the Latin (Western) tradition and the Greek (Eastern) tradition. One could ask what happened to the Syrian tradition, which was one among several in the East. Silence in response to this question is a common answer.

Most presentations and programs of study concentrate their efforts on the Latin and Greek branches, so a *tertium non datur* is never mentioned as a general reference, as excellently phrased by Sebastian Brock:

> Such a dichotomy is both unfortunate and inadequate, for it completely overlooks the existence of the oriental Christian Churches which constitute an important third stream of Christian Tradition, quite distinct from the other two familiar streams. Among the Oriental Christian Churches those within the Syriac liturgical tradition may be said to hold pride and place, since they are representatives of, and to some degree direct heirs to, Semitic world out of which Christianity sprang.[1]

Part of the forgotten richness of the third stream are the writings of Aphrahat, Ephrem, Evagrius of Pontus, Abraham of Nathpar, Isaac of Nineveh, and John of Apamea. One of the most significant motivations for this research was the need to rediscover this *tertium non datur* in many handbooks of Christian tradition. Among the aforementioned authors, John of Apamea is one of the most intriguing figures because of the mystery and confusion that surrounds his historical identity. This Syrian personage also wrote extensively, and his writings are replete with profound theological and spiritual reflections that made him famous in antiquity.

As deduced from previous comments, the present work is developed in two major parts. The first part expounds the problem related to the quest of identifying the historical John of Apamea, a Syrian Monk who became famous for his spiritual and theological writings. Thus the investigation presents an overview of the problem of his identity based upon the most important critical works attributed to him in order to propose a possible solution to the quest for the historical John of Apamea. Among the scholarly and critical editions of his oeuvre, it is worth mentioning in this introduction the work published in 1936 by Sven

1 Cf. Sebastian Brock, *The Syriac Fathers on Prayer and the Spiritual Life* (Kalamazoo, MI: Cistercian Publications Inc., 1987), x.

Dedering entitled "Ein Dialog über die Seele und die Affekte des Menschen."[2] This volume presents four dialogues accredited to John regarding the soul and passions of a human person. Those writings became well-known in antiquity because they describe the most famous anthropological tripartite conception of body, soul, and spirit which is based on Pauline theology (cf. 1Thess 5:23) and becomes one of the most well known notions in the theological thought of this Syrian spiritual father. But, is this notion present in all his works? Is it truly the most important anthropological conception of the Solitary monk?

In the analysis of these critical editions, this present research takes a critical approach towards the generalization of the tripartite notion, since it cannot be found in the other writings attributed to the Syrian monk. In order to demonstrate the inadequacy of this generalization, I will present a summary of the second and sixth dialogue of John of Apamea with Thomasios, within which are concentrated the theological and spiritual notions of the Solitary monk that are contained explicitly or implicitly in most of the *opus* now attributed to him. For this reason I will also present an analytical summary regarding the oeuvre of John the Solitary of Apamea through the publications of Lars Gösta Rignell, Werner Strothmann, Irenée Hausherr, Jean-Claude Guy, Ortíz de Urbina, and René Lavenant.

A summary of the content of the second and sixth dialogue with Thomasios is also presented in this section as an illustration of theological evidence in order to prove and establish that the most general theological notion of John is the dualistic conception of the world and the human person (anthropological conception). The summary of the dialogues is faithful to the critical editions of Lavenant and Strothmann, but does not pretend to be a literal translation of the Syriac text. I could not use an English critical translation from the Syriac text in my research because such a critical or official translation for all six dialogues with Thomasios does not exist.

John of Apamea elucidates in his dialogues with Thomasios several different theological ideas, among which the Eschatological dimension receives a place of preeminence. However, another center of his theological thought is widely examined under the notion of the spiritual and corporeal senses used by the interior and exterior person to know and experience the realities of the present world (material experience) and the world to come (spiritual experience and knowledge). The expression "spiritual sense" is *per se* a paradox, since the spirit, by its proper essence, subsists independently from the body and from the sensorial means that the body needs to interact dynamically with the surrounding

---

2 Cf. Johannes von Lycopolis, *Ein Dialog über die Seele und die Affekte des Menschen*, ed. et trans., Sven Dedering (Leipzig – Uppsala – Haag: Harrassowitz Verlag, 1936).

world. It is important to affirm that John of Apamea does not reject the physical world and the corporeal senses. He sees in the present world an opportunity to develop the spiritual senses through exercise and a process of purification in order to perceive the divine reality immersed in the circumstantial reality.

The notion of the spiritual perception of the soul is also intrinsically connected with the idea and practice of "spiritual exegesis." This kind of methodological approach to the Scripture has been extensively developed since the third century, especially in the School of Alexandria which was the cultural milieu of formation for the Syrian monk.

The second part of the investigation concentrates on the specific topic of *spiritual seeing* in Mark's Gospel. This section follows four methodological stages derived from the notions of the spiritual perception according to the theology of John of Apamea. The first consists in the semantic analysis of the terminology employed by the author of Mark according to the Greek text presented by Nestle–Aland 28th edition. The semantic clarification is complemented by examining the psychological approach implied in the categories of *seeing* and *seeing as*. The act of *seeing* an object or event can be real regardless of whether the object or event of sight is by nature tangible or intangible for other observers. This aspect gives psychological (or scientific) support to the notion of spiritual seeing as an act that can be real even though the reality perceived by the person of faith cannot be witnessed by other persons.

The second stage analyzes the portrait of the seeing of Jesus in the narrative. This is the portion of the investigation that moves from the literal sense to the spiritual sense implied in the Markan narrative. The selected pericopes portray characteristics of the seeing of Christ that express the theological intention and originality of the author. Following the same methodological path, the third stage briefly examines the attitude and seeing of the demons in the accounts of exorcism by exposing their unique behavioral pattern. The last stage considers the narrative portrait given in the contemplative attitude of the women in the context of the crucifixion and burial of Jesus as an instance of purely spiritual seeing.

The study of the biblical texts embodies a multidimensional world. The Historical-critical approach to the Scripture has devoted decades to discovering the *world behind the sacred text*. The life setting in which the text was produced is crucial in order to understand the theological intention of the real author who was writing to a real audience. In more recent times, exegetical approaches try to expose the *world in the text*, which present the characteristics and theology of the texts in their final form. The canonical text, namely, the sacred text in its final written stage, transmits linguistic and theological dimensions that surpass the historical limitations in which it was born, acquiring an independent life of its own and becoming a source of theology and spirituality for the generations to come.[3] Contemporary critics have been dedicating more attention to *the world in front of the text*. This dimension emphasizes the narratological category of the text for the reader in front of whom the sacred text is presented as a piece of art that was composed in order to be admired and interpreted by an audience. This is one of many technical nuances proper to narrative criticism, a method that has been acquiring an increasing amount of interest in the field of biblical scholarship.[4] The second part of this investigation predominantly applies this approach of narrative analysis to the sacred text of Mark as a *locus theologicus*, taking the canonical text in its final form as the object of study which is, at the same time, a source of theological richness. The results of the synchronic approach are complemented with some of the results provided by the diachronic studies that help the reader to comprehend more readily the intention and theology of the actual author of Mark's Gospel.

The Greek koiné presents a wide spectrum of terms utilized to signify the notion of seeing. Among the rich terminology employed in this *Wortfeld*, it is possible to identify three important verbs that signify visual perception: Horáō, Blépō, and Theōréō, each with their respective nuances in Mark's Gospel. In addition to their lexicographic definitions, they also acquire a very unique semantic dimension depending on their syntactic subject, object, and context in the narrative. These syntactic determinations of the narrative criticism applied to selected pericopes allow the reader to discover a metaphysical portrait of seeing in Jesus, demons, and the women. The reading of the metaphysical portrait in the Gospel finds its hermeneutical ground in the notion of the senses of the soul developed by Origen and the Alexandrian Tradition and later elaborated upon in the theological thought of John of Apamea. Such a notion will also find an important development in its practical application to the field of the spiritual exercises of Ignatius of Loyola. This hermeneutical reading applied to the Markan pericopes through the narrative and semantic approach helps the reader to discover the spiritual dimension of the visual perception of the personages of Jesus, the demons, and the women.

---

3 Cf. John N. Oswalt, "Canonical Criticism: A Review From A Conservative Viewpoint," *JETS* 30/3 (1987): 318; James Barr, "Childs' Introduction to the Old Testament as scripture," *JSOT* 16 (1980): 16; Brevard S. Childs, "The Canonical Shape of the Prophetic Literature," *Interpretation* 32 (1978): 53; John H. Sailhamer, *Introduction to Old Testament Theology: A Canonical Approach* (Grand Rapids: Zondervan, 1995), 97-103.

4 Cf. Mark A. Powell, *What is Narrative Criticism?* (Minneapolis: Fortress Press 1990); Sandra M. Schneiders, *The Revelatory Text. Interpreting the New Testament as Sacred Scripture* (San Franciso: Harper, 1991); James Resseguie, *Narrative Criticism of the New Testament* (Grand Rapids: Baker Academic, 2005).

The semantic implications in the context of visual perception in the kerygmatic narrative provide a pragmatic dimension that is addressed to the community implied in the Markan narrative. The real and implicit audience of the Gospel is impelled to adopt the portrait of seeing which the author wishes them to have. One of the intentions of the kerygmatic story of the Gospel is to motivate its audience to adopt and implement the spiritual seeing of Jesus in their personal lives. Thus there is a pragmatic dimension implied in the Markan narrative that can be gleaned from the semantic implications of the verbs of visual perception, encouraging the audience to adopt the manner of seeing which the author deems best. When the audience (implied or real) assumes as part of their spiritual behavior the seeing of Jesus, they are incarnating and exemplifying the seeing of God. Thus the message of the Gospel goes beyond the historical limits of its original receptors, becoming a spiritual model and foundation that motivates a true experience of faith in the reader who approaches the inspired text to find the living word of God in this present world.

Part One

John of Apamea and His Oeuvre

Chapter I

John of Apamea's Writings and Identity

1. Premise: Eastern Christianity

The Eastern Christian church during the second and third centuries had been manifesting the same fluctuations in prosperity and decadence that can be observed in the Western Church that was attached to the Roman Empire. However, during the fourth and fifth centuries, the barbarian invasions radically changed the history of Western civilization with the end of the Roman Empire, transforming the history of Christianity in the hemisphere. The same fate did not befall the Byzantine Empire, promoting prosperity in the fields of literature and culture and enabling the Eastern Church to flourish in matters of theology with its high speculative elucidations. Then Eastern Christianity centered its theology on a more metaphysical and speculative approach, while the Western church distinguished itself through more practical, hierarchical, and devotional aspects of theology.[1]

Among the diverse literal and cultural manifestations found in the Eastern Christian communities, there appeared without doubt two main distinct centers of theological reflection with their respective methodological lines: the Alexandrian and the Antiochian schools of theology. The former followed a platonic philosophical path of reflection that was manifested in its tendency to cultivate a more spiritual and mystic theology, accompanied by an allegorical and symbolic exegesis of Scripture. Among the prominent figures of this current of theology were Athanasius,[2] Origen,[3] the three Cappadocian Fathers—Basil the Great,[4]

---

1 Cf. Bernardino Llorca, Ricardo García-Villoslada, and Juan María Laboa, *Historia de la Iglesia Católica* (Madrid: BAC, 1996), I, 580-581.

2 Cf. PG 25-28.

3 Since the work of Origen is monumental, I indicate only some of his works translated into English: Origen, *On John's Gospel*, ed. A. E. Brooke (Cambridge: Cambridge Uni-

Gregory the Theologian (or Gregory Nazianzen),[5] and Gregory of Nyssa[6]—Cyril of Alexandria,[7] and Pseudo-Dionysius the Areopagite,[8] among others. The school of Antioch, on the other hand, followed the traits of Aristotelian philosophy, expressed in its realistic theology that highlighted the human aspect of Christology, accompanied with a more literal and philological exegetical study of Scripture. The Antiochian school also had outstanding theologians who were prominent thinkers and models of sanctity in antiquity. Among its more prominent figures were John Chrysostom,[9] Theodoret of Cyrrhus,[10] Diodorus of Tarso,[11] and Theodore of Mopsuestia.[12]

Both schools, because of their respective methodological paths, fell into extreme positions many times, producing some deviations from true Christian orthodoxy in different historical periods. Between these two theological schools, there emerged a rivalry that eventually forced the production of a new vocabulary and reflections that helped to shape the comprehension and formulations of the dogmas concerning the Christological and Trinitarian aspects of the hypo-

---

versity Press, 1896), I-II; Id., *C. Cels.*, trans. Henry Chadwick (Cambridge: Cambridge University Press, 1965); Id., *Contre Celse*, trans. Marcel Borrett, SC 147(Paris: Les Éditions du Cerf 1969); Id., "On First Principles," trans. G. W. Butterworth (Gloucester, MA: Peter Smith, 1973); Id., *An Exhortation to Martyrdom; Prayer; First Principles, Book IV; Prologue to the Commentary on the Song of Songs; Homily XXVII on Numbers*, trans. R. Greer (Classics of Western Spirituality; New York: Paulist Press, 1979); Id., *Homilies on Genesis and Exodus*, trans. R.E. Heine (Washington, DC: Catholic University of America, 1982); Id., *Commentary on the Gospel According to John, Books 1-10*, trans. R.E. Heine (Washington, DC: Catholic University of America, 1989).

4 Cf. PG 29-32.

5 Cf. PG 35-38.

6 Cf. PG 44-46.

7 Cf. PG 68-77.

8 Cf. PG 3-4.

9 Cf. PG 47-64.

10 Cf. PG 80-84. Regarding a publication of his works, see Gerard H. Ettlinger, *Theodoret: Eranistes* (Washington, DC: Catholic University of America Press, 2003); John F. Petruccione and Robert C. Hill, *Theodoret of Cyrus. The Questions on the Octateuch* (Greek text and English translation; Washington, DC: Catholic University of America Press, 2007); István Pásztori-Kupán, *Theodoret of Cyrus. The Early Church Fathers* (London, New York: Routledge, 2006). Includes full translations of "On the Trinity," "On the Incarnation," and excerpts from "A Cure of Greek Maladies" and "A Compendium of Heretical Mythification."

11 Cf. PG 33.

12 Cf. PG 66.

static union, the natures and the wills of the person of Christ, and other dogmatic debates.

Among the Eastern theological writings, of special importance is the Syrian Christian literature that began to be developed in the fourth century in Mesopotamia and its surrounding areas. One of the first and most worthwhile manifestations of Syrian writing can be found in the "Acta Martyrum" of the great Christian persecution in Persia during the fourth century;[13] however, the most significant representatives of Syrian Christian literature during the fourth century were Aphraates († 345 CE) and Ephrem the Syrian († 373 CE).

Aphraates[14] was an ascetic monk who became a Bishop. He was a prominent theologian and spiritual father who attained fame because of his erudition, and for that reason he was also known as the "wise monk." The writings of Aphraates, as we know them, consist of twenty-three "Demonstrations," or homilies on the moral and ascetic life. Among the most essential spiritual and theological themes treated by Aphraates we find Faith, Charity, the real presence of the Body and Blood of Christ in the Eucharist, the perpetual virginity of the Blessed Virgin and her Divine Maternity, the foundation of the Church on the apostle Peter, the existence of the sacraments (except matrimony, which is not mentioned by him in his writings), Fasting, Prayer, Wars, Monks, Penitents, Resurrection, and Humility. The value of these theological and moral tractates consist in their portrayal of theology, Christian history and faith of the Syrian communities in antiquity which was in agreement to the faith manifested in Nicea (325 CE).

The most prominent theologian of that century in the Syrian tradition in general was Ephrem, who reveals in his writings the summit of Syrian literature.[15] Born around the year 306 in the city of Nisibis—the modern Turkish town

13 Cf. Llorca, García-Villoslada, and Laboa, *Historia*, 468.

14 Cf. Llorca, García-Villoslada, and Laboa, *Historia*, 468-469. Regarding the works of Aphraates, see Rubens Duval, *La littérature syriaque* (Paris: V. Lacoffre, 1900), 224-229; Jérôme Labourt, *Le christianisme dans l'empire perse sous la dynastie Sassanide* (Bibliotheque de l'enseignement de l'histoire ecclesiastique; Paris: V. Lecoffre, ^{2}1904); Alphonse Mingana, *Sources syriaques* (Leipzig,: Harrassowitz Verlag, 1907), I-II; William Wright, *The homilies of Aphraates, the* Persian sage. Vol. I. The Syriac text (London,: Williams and Norgate, 1869).

15 See Andrew Palmer, "A Single Human Being Divided in Himself: Ephraim the Syrian, the Man in the Middle," *Hugoye*: *Journal of Syriac Studies* 1, no. 2 (1998): 119-163; Id., "The Influence of Ephraim the Syrian," *Hugoye*: *Journal of Syriac Studies* 2, no. 1 (1999): 83-109; Hannah M. Hunt, "The Tears of the Sinful Woman: A Theology of Redemption in the Homilies of St. Ephraim and his Followers," *Hugoye*: *Journal of Syriac Studies* 1, no. 2 (1998): 165-184; Sidney H. Griffith, "A Spiritual Father for the Whole

of Nusaybin—in the Roman province of Mesopotamia, he became a theologian with exceptional erudition. As the head of the School of Edessa, he led it to the summit of its abundant theological fruitfulness. Because of his great humility, Ephrem never accepted the position of a bishop, which was offered to him on more than one occasion. This aspect of his meek personality continued to be manifested in his personal sense of inadequacy for the priesthood, which led him to live as a deacon for the rest of his life, not asking or looking for positions in the ecclesiastical hierarchy. Through his life of consecration, his reputation as a great theologian, orator, ascetic, and poet grew and spread throughout the Eastern Church, to the point that he was given the nickname "cithara of the Holy Spirit."[16] Among his numerous writings known to us, only a few works have been preserved in Syriac, Greek, Armenian, and Coptic. He wrote commentaries on almost all the books of the Scripture, but only the commentaries in Syriac on the books of Genesis, Exodus, and Paralipomenon (Chronicles) survived. He also wrote biblical commentaries on Tatian's Diatessaron, the Acts of the Apostles, and the Pauline Epistles, which are preserved in Armenian. His exegetical methodology was built upon a literal study of the text and accompanied by mystical and allegorical interpretations, finding a good balance between these two hermeneutical approaches. When we take into consideration his dogmatic writings, his fifty sermons against Gnostics, his discourses on the feasts of the Lord and the saints, the moral tractates, and his ascetic poetry known by the title of *Carmina Nisibena*,[17] all hold positions of prominence. One of the most noteworthy characteristics of Ephrem's writings is his poetic and semi-poetic form of writing theology that combines the beauty of the grammatical expression with the profound sense of the spiritual and theological elucidations about God and humankind.

The legacy of Ephrem continued among his disciples in the Syrian and Armenian currents of theology. One of his prominent disciples in the Syrian tradition was the abbot of a monastery in Antioch known as Isaac the Great († 460 CE). In the collection at the monastery were found publications of his works composed in metric verse regarding moral and theological themes.[18] Other important agents of this theological path were Mesrop († 441 CE), who can be considered the father of the Christian literature in Armenian, and Eznik of Kolb (†

Church: The Universal Appeal of St. Ephraem the Syrian," *Hugoye*: *Journal of Syriac Studies* 1, no. 2 (1998): 197-220.

16 Cf. Llorca, García-Villoslada, and Laboa, *Historia*, 469.

17 Ibidem.

18 See Paul Bedjan, *Homiliae S. Isaaci Syri Antiocheni* (Paris – Leipzig: Harrassowitz Verlag, 1903), I; Id., *Mar Isaacus Ninivita. De Perfectione Religiosa* (Paris – Leipzig: Harrassowitz Verlag, 1909).

ca. 450 CE), the Bishop of Bagrevand, who was a faithful disciple of his holy master, Mesrop, and continued his theology. With Eznik, Armenian Christian literature achieved great prosperity. Among his writings, it is significant to mention his *Refutatio contra Sectam*, which was a solid expression of Christian apologetics, giving a rational and spiritual basis for the Christian faith.[19]

The legacy of the Syrian theology continued with a great variety of authors and thinkers. The monks of the time present a good example, for they cultivated the practical dimension of their mystical life with theological and abstract reflections of their divine contemplations. Some of these mystical theologians were better known than others in past centuries. Among these unknown authors of the Syrian tradition, however, one can find many jewels of Christian literature, expressed in delicate spiritual and theological elucidations, as in the case of the writings of the solitary monks who followed the same traditions of mysticism, morality, and theology expressed splendidly by Ephrem.

Evidence has been found of the first manifestations of "monastic" life in Egypt and the surrounding areas in the East since the end of the first century and the beginning of the second. By the fifth century, Egypt had become something of a monastic dream world shaped by the eastern ideals of the monastic life.[20] Many people felt the need to live the *Xeniteia* by practicing Christianity in a more rigid and austere manner, eliminating any possible worldly distractions in their path of *synousia*, or communication and union with God. *Xeniteia* was "the voluntary alienation by which ascetics sought release from material and social circumstances that might hinder their ability to trust in God and make spiritual progress."[21] This way of life was an attempt to achieve a faithful observation of the evangelical beatitudes through nonparticipation in vain pleasures, abstention from matrimony, and a severe practice of penance and piety, factors considered essential to live a life of perfect asceticism. Those who consecrated themselves to this kind of life were called "solitaries" or *anachoretae* (ἀναχωρητῄς) because they lived isolated from everyone, avoiding any kind of community.[22] Beginning in the fourth century, this solitary kind of life became increasingly popular in the eastern churches, especially those of Syrian-speaking communities. The growth of spiritual Christian fervor was escalating among men and women looking for a closer relationship with the Lord. Many of these "solitaries" wrote extensively, including letters, dialogues, and tractates of pro-

19 Cf. Llorca, García-Villoslada, and Laboa, *Historia*, 586.

20 Cf. Daniel Caner, *Wandering, Begging Monks. Spiritual Authority and the Promotion of Monasticism in Late Antiquity* (Berkeley – Los Angeles – London, UK: University of California Press, 2002), 20.

21 Daniel Caner, *Wandering, Begging Monks*, 25.

22 Cf. BAGD, "ἀναχωρέω," 63.

found theological and mystical values and acquired great reputations of holiness. Among these anchorites, we center our attention on John of Apamea, also known as John the Solitary (īḥīdāyā), since he was one of those extraordinary people who wanted to achieve the perfect mystic life. The problem with this Syrian author resides in the lack of information about him, a difficulty that leads us first to deal with the quest for his historical identity, triggered by the classification and authorship of writings attributed—or not ascribed—to him. Making use of this methodological starting point, I would like to construct some aspects of his theology, anthropology, and mystical principles that can serve as reading tools to interpret the visual perception in Mark's Gospel.

2. The Translated and Edited Works of John of Apamea

Between 1922 and 1965, Anton Baumstark and Ignacio Ortíz de Urbina[23] proposed in their respective studies John the Solitary of Apamea as the correct author of a series of ascetic tractates and dialogues that have been preserved in Syriac since 581 CE. One of the first critical editions of the work of John of Apamea, however, appeared in 1936, published by Sven Dedering under the title *Ein Dialog über die Seele und die Affekte des Menschen*,[24] a dialogue about the soul and the passions of men.[25] This edition included a set of four dialogues and an exposition regarding the problem of the authorship of the text, for Dedering attributed the writings to a so-called John of Lycopolis, also known as John of Egypt, the seer of Thebaid, a renowned ascetic who died in Thebaid circa 394 CE.[26] With his study, Dedering undertook the task of solving the mysterious puzzle surrounding the authorship of the four dialogues on the soul and human passions. It was not until Irenée Hausherr presented strict scrutiny and research in the introduction of his French translation of the *Dialogue sur l'âme et les pas-*

23 Cf. Anton Baumstark, *Geschichte der syrischen Literatur: Mit Ausschluss der christlich-palästinensischen Texte* (Bonn: A. Markus und E. Webers Verlag, 1922), 88-90; Ignacio Ortíz de Urbina, *Patrologia syriaca* (Roma: Pontificio Institutum Orientalium Studiorum, 1965), 109.

24 Cf. Johannes von Lycopolis, *Ein Dialog über die Seele und die Affekte des Menschen*, ed. et trans. Sven Dedering (Leipzig – Uppsala – Haag: Harrassowitz Verlag, 1936).

25 The term "men" in this translation of "Menschen" incorporates all humankind: male and female.

26 This ascetic monk was contemporary to John of Apamea, and the writings attributed to him are disputed. Cf. Jean D'Apamée, *Dialogues et Traités*, ed. et trans. René Lavenant, Introduction, traduction et notes, Sources Chrétiennes 311 (Paris: Les Éditions du Cerf, 1984), 15; Jean-Claude Guy, "Jean de Lycopolis," *DSAM* VI, 619-620.

sions des homes[27] that these dialogues were attributed to John of Apamea. With this proposal, a new platform was established for a more accurate approach in the historical discovery of this worthy but unknown Christian author.[28]

With Hausherr's contribution, the problem of the person of John of Apamea became evident. According to his historical research, the existence of several monks in antiquity who had the same name and were practicing an eremitic and ascetic lifestyle in the solitude of the desert in Egypt, Syria, and Mesopotamia has been attested. Therefore, the crucial question is which monk was the responsible for the Syrian writings in the published works mentioned above. Was there another author among the group of ascetics who was also named John? Which John among the group of ascetics is the John known as John of Apamea?

A notable example of this problem, as René Lavenant presents it, is the publication of three letters in 1941 that were attributed to John the Solitary by Lars Gösta Rignell.[29] The second letter contains a passage that is already known in other documents because it was quoted by a Nestorian monk called Babai the Great (circa 551–628 CE), who ascribed the statement to John the Solitary from the land of Apamea.[30] Based on this information, the chronological life setting of the author generates questions that provoke more debate and elucidations because, if this "John" is the same person who is responsible both for the dialogue edited by Sven Dedering and the three letters edited by Rignell, the reader must locate the author and his writings between the second half of the fourth century and the first half of the sixth century, possibly even the first two decades of the seventh century. This problem was addressed previously by Hausherr, who presented his proposal of multiple authors to resolve the problem of John's identity. Nevertheless, Rignell went on in 1960 to publish another three tractates about spiritual perfection and baptism attributed to John of Apamea titled *Drei Traktate von Johannes dem Einsiedler*, which can be translated as "Three Trac-

---

27 Cf. Jean le Solitaire (Pseudo-Jean de Lycopolis), *Dialogue sur l'âme et les passions des homes*, ed. et trans. Irenée Hausherr Traduit du syriaque sur l'edition de Sven Dedering, Orientalia Christiana Analecta 120 (Roma: Pontificio Institutum Orientalium Studiorum, 1939). See also Lavenant, *Dialogues*, 15.

28 Cf. Irenée Hausherr, "Un grand auteur spirituel retrouvé: Jean d'Apamée," *OCP* 14 (1948): 3-42.

29 Lars Gösta Rignell, ed., *Briefe von Johannes dem Einsiedler mit kritischem Apparat, Einleitung und Übersetzung*, (Lund: Håkan Ohlssons Boktryckeri, 1941); Lavenant, *Dialogues*, 16.

30 Cf. Rignell, *Briefe*, 80, 18-84, 4.

tates of John the Hermit." However, in Rignell's work, the problem of the authorship persisted.[31]

Another important illustration of the problem is provided by William Cureton, who in his *Corpus Ignatianum* published a letter from a monk called John the monk, the seer of Thebaid, to Eutropius and Eusebius: *Epistula ad Eutropium et Eusebium de communione veritatis in vita nova* (Ms Add 12170, fol. 211).[32] The author of this letter, according to the cross-references with other collected documents obtained from William Wright[33] and *Corpus Ignatianum*,[34] can be dated between the eighth and ninth centuries.[35] Other works carrying the name of John the monk appear in several Syriac manuscripts in the British Museum, as shown in Wright's Catalogue,[36] among which are preserved other letters addressed to the same monks, Eutropius and Eusebius. The complexity of the identification of the author called "John" becomes more evident in the Ms Add 17169,[37] where a document bearing the authorship of "John, the Monk" is dated circa 581 CE.[38] Therefore, there are catalogued and published documents attributed to "John, the solitary monk from Thebaid" that can be dated between the sixth and ninth centuries. The extensive period over which documents were accredited to a so-called "John, the Monk" has stimulated research to discover the true identity of the solitary monk known in the orthodox Syrian tradition as John of Apamea.

In 1972, Werner Strothmann edited six dialogues, two letters, and three tractates, all of which he attributed to John of Apamea.[39] Strothmann used the name of "John" with different classifications, but in the end, he always referred to a Syrian monk called John the Solitary from Apamea in Syria. These writings have the major theological themes of hope in the resurrection, God's economy of salvation manifested in Christ, the spiritual path that includes the notions of

31 Cf. Johannes von Apamea, *Drei Traktate von Johannes dem Einsiedler*, ed. et trans. Lars Gösta Rignell (Lund: C.W.K. Gleerup, 1960).

32 Cf. William Cureton, *Corpus Ignatianum.* A Complete Collection (Berlin: Asher and Co., 1849), 351.

33 Cf. William Wright, *Catalogue of Syriac Manuscripts* (London: British Museum of Oriental Printed Books and Manuscripts, 1838, 1870), 749-767.

34 Cf. Cureton, *Corpus Ignatianum*, 205. 239-240.

35 Cf. Joseph B. Lightfoot, *The Apostolic Fathers* (Hildesheim – Zürich – New York: Georg Olms 1890, 1973), II/1, 153.

36 Cf. Wright, *Catalogue*, 1296.

37 Cf. Wright, *Catalogue*, 451.

38 Cf. Lightfoot, *The Apostolic Fathers*, 153.

39 Werner Strothmann, *Johannes vom Apamea, Sechs Gespräche mit Thomasios, Der Briefewechsel zwischen Thomasios und Johannes und drei an Thomasios gerichtete Abhandlungen*, Patristische Texte und Studien 11 (Berlin: Walter de Gruyter, 1972).

the superior invisible senses of the soul, and the obstacles of the present corporeal world. The value of this German translation from the Syriac resides in the historical and doctrinal research concerning the figure of John of Apamea.

René Lavenant, using Strothmann's contribution regarding the historical quest for John of Apamea, produced a noteworthy critical introduction to the *disputatio* surrounding the writings attributed to the Syrian anchorite, presenting an acclaimed translation of some of his writings from Syriac. In a scholarly manner, Lavenant engages the historical problem of the person of John of Apamea from Syria by attributing to him the six dialogues with Thomasios, two letters, and three tractates published in 1984.[40]

A reader today can find the edited works attributed to John of Apamea by Strothmann[41] and Lavenant in German and French. However, the acquisition of these works is very difficult because they have been out of print for at least fifteen years; furthermore, critical editions in English based upon the Syrian texts have not yet been published, making this field of study difficult to learn about the theological insights and personality of the Syrian spiritual father. Such obstacles are the reason behind the present investigation, which aims to make these literary and spiritual jewels, buried for centuries, accessible to a wider audience of readers.

The following précis provides an overview of the published works of John of Apamea divided into three categories: dialogues, letters, and tractates.

The dialogues with Thomasios are as follows:

a) The *First Dialogue with* Thomasios addresses the hope for the future of the world to come.[42]

b) The *Second Dialogue with Thomasios* explains the transformation that will benefit humankind in the future, specifying that the future world will be spiritual. In this dialogue, the reader explicitly faces the doctrine of the senses of the soul as understood by John of Apamea.[43]

c) The *Third Dialogue with Thomasios* deals with the creation of human beings and why every person has been created to receive a divine destiny in the world

40 Cf. Lavenant, *Dialogues*, 27.

41 Cf. Strothmann, *Johannes vom Apamea*, 45-56.

42 Cf. Johannes vom Apamea, *Gespräche* 1, 1–13; Strothmann, *Johannes vom Apamea*, 116-122.

43 Cf. Johannes vom Apamea, *Gespräche* 2, 13–21; Strothmann, *Johannes vom Apamea*, 123-127.

to come. The topics of discussion are the nature of angels, cherubs, and seraphim and the composite nature of the human body.[44]

d) The *Fourth Dialogue with Thomasios* explicates the theme of the extreme variety of beings created by God in the natural world and outside of physical nature. In this conversation, John compares the physical and the spiritual world.[45]

e) The *Fifth Dialogue with Thomasios* analyzes the issue of the composite human body and how a process of purification is an indispensable path that leads to a transformation that elevates the human soul above the natural world to receive the benefits of the spiritual world of God.[46]

f) The *Sixth Dialogue with Thomasios* addresses the revelations and visions of the divine economy of salvation in this present world and the salutary economy of the world to come. Here, the author also employs the notion of the spiritual senses as the perceptive means (physical and spiritual) to know the spiritual realities and the mysteries of God.[47]

The two letters mentioned in this present study are published in the critical editions of Strothmann and Lavenant who, in agreement, accredited them to John of Apamea. The letters are as follows:

a) The *first letter* from master John to Thomasios speaks of faith as the only tool that Christians have to approach the mystery of the divine economy of Christ. Faith is presented as the perfect instrument to know divine realities.[48]

b) The *second letter* is from Thomasios to his master, John of Apamea. This brief epistle is concerned with the proper explanations that a disciple requires from his master regarding the universal dimension of Christ's mystery of salvation, and what the proper attitude would be in relation to this mystery of salvation.[49]

---

44 Cf. Johannes vom Apamea, *Gespräche* 3, 22–35; Strothmann, *Johannes vom Apamea*, 128-136.

45 Cf. Johannes vom Apamea, *Gespräche* 4, 36–58; Strothmann, *Johannes vom Apamea*, 137-150.

46 Cf. Johannes vom Apamea, *Gespräche* 5, 59–69; Strothmann, *Johannes vom Apamea*, 151-156.

47 Cf. Johannes vom Apamea, *Gespräche* 6, 70–81; Strothmann, *Johannes vom Apamea*, 157-164.

48 Cf. Johannes vom Apamea, *Briefe* 82–90; Strothmann, *Johannes vom Apamea*, 165-169.

49 Cf. Johannes vom Apamea, *Briefe* 90–93; Strothmann, *Johannes vom Apamea*, 170-171.

The three tractates embody theological essays that cannot be understood as a systematic dissertation using the terms of our modern theological conceptions. The tractates correspond to spiritual expositions that deal with Trinitarian, Eschatological, Christological, and anthropological notions, functioning as the platform to elucidate the mysteries implied in the salutary history of mankind according to the divine economy. What follows are very brief summaries identifying the main themes of each tractate.

a) The *first tractate* shows the perfection and universality in the notions of time and space in the person, action, and teachings of Jesus Christ.[50]

b) The *second tractate* provides responses to questions regarding the incarnation of Christ, the combat between Christ and Satan when He was tempted in the desert, and the great mystery of suffering on the Cross.[51]

c) The *third tractate* addresses the great cosmic and universal dimension of Christ. The *Logos* (Jesus Christ) is the beginning, the middle, and the end of every cosmic and universal movement of salvation. Through him, God establishes a very special relationship with humanity until the end of this present world and the complete manifestation of God's world — or the divine reality — in all its complexity. In this salutary dimension, Christ is the only hope for humanity.[52]

Ebedjesu also gives a list of works accredited to John of Apamea: "tres composuit tomos, necnon epistolas, de Regimine Spirituali, de Passionibus, et de Perfectione."[53] In Wright's Catalogue appears the Letter to Eutropios and Eusebius on the spiritual life.[54] In 1987, Sebastian Brock was the first scholar to publish "The Letter to Hesychius," which was attributed to John of Apamea. Regarding this document, Brock affirms:

> The identity of Hesychius is not known, but on internal grounds it is clear that he had only recently adopted the monastic life. John's Letter provides him with much practical advice. An indication of how greatly this advice was appreciated by later

50 Cf. Jean D'Apamée, *Traité* 1, 94–113; Lavenant, *Dialogues*, 130-145.

51 Cf. Jean D'Apamée, *Traité* 2, 113–126; Lavenant, *Dialogues*, 146-157.

52 Cf. Jean D'Apamée, *Traité* 3, 126–141; Lavenant, *Dialogues*, 158-170.

53 Georgius Ebedjesu Khayyath, *Syri Orientales, seu Chaldaei, Nestoriani et Romanorum Pontificum Primatus. Commentatio Historico-philologico-theologica.* Syriac Studies Library 105 (Piscataway, NJ: Gorgias Press, 1870, 2011), III, 50.

54 Cf. Wright, *Catalogue*, 451.657.

generations of monks is given by the large number of manuscripts which survive containing the Letter.[55]

Through my research, I have encountered a variety of writings (*opera*) that can be credited with a respectable degree of probability to John of Apamea. It is worthwhile to indicate that these works are unpublished, or if they have been published, a report about them as such in works and publications revised within the last seventy years does not exist. For this reason, in line with the research of Strothmann, Lavenant, van Leijsen, and the review of the Syriac Catalogues of Wright and Cureton, I consider it important to indicate in this section of the investigation that there are unpublished or unreported works of John of Apamea.[56] These include:

a) The first tractate regarding the new world.
b) The second tractate about the new world.
c) The accomplishment of the divine promises in the future and the new life.
d) A writing that tries to answer the question of why in this world good people are miserable and unhappy and wicked people are happy and fortunate.
e) The first tractate about the end of the world.
f) The second tractate about the end of the world, which includes a doxology.
g) A letter to Eubule.

Currently, there are three lost works of John of Apamea, according to Strothmann and Lavenant.[57] They are as follows:

a) A work on the nature of demons.
b) A work on the Epiphany of the Lord.
c) Hymns.

3. The Identity of John of Apamea: Proposals

A brief overview of the writings attributed to John of Apamea gives the reader glimpses into the issue of the chronological setting of this figure in history. In considering a collection of letters, dialogues, tractates, and quotations from other well-known personages of the Eastern Church, the resulting time frame covers a period that extends from the second half of the fourth century until the first half of the seventh century. This chronological setting, which would be quite a

55 Brock, *The Syriac Fathers*, 79. The Letter to Hesychius is contained in pages 81-98.

56 Cf. Strothmann, *Gespräche*, 61; Lavenant, *Dialogues*, 27. For a summary of the undisputed and disputed works of John of Apamea, see L. van Leijsen, "De driedeling van het geestelijk leven bij Johannes van Apamea. Kritische kanttekeningen bij enige gangbare interpretaties," *JECS* 51, no. 3-4 (1999): 213-240.

57 Cf. Strothmann, *Gespräche*, 56; Lavenant, *Dialogues*, 27.

stretch for the lifespan of one person, leads to the problem of the identity of the so-called "John the Solitary from Apamea."

Proposals made by scholars such as Strothmann, Hausherr, Baumstark, and Lavenant became tentative solutions concerning the authenticity and identity of this Syrian monk, who is considered the author of significant theological and spiritual writings. In this regard, it is valuable to assert that John had an illustrious reputation among the monks in Palestine from whom Thomasios heard about him, after which he did not hesitate to travel to the land of Apamea to meet and learn from this master of spirituality.[58]

Taking into consideration the criterion of the identity of the monk in relation to the published works previously presented, the proposals can be classified into three main groups:

a) The proposal of three different persons
b) The proposal of two different persons
c) The proposal of one John of Apamea

At this point, the next step is a succinct examination of each theory.

3.1. The Hypothesis of Three Different Persons

The most representative scholars of this hypothesis are Hausherr and Lavenant, who proposed the distinction of three different persons, all with the name "John of Apamea."[59] The first John of Apamea, the author of the aforementioned six dialogues, two letters, and three tractates, was from Syria. This John existed within a period spanning from the second half of the fourth century until the first half of the fifth century. He can be classified as the Proto-John of Apamea,[60] and according to the reconstruction proposed by Lavenant, the *terminus ad quem* to determine the period in which he lived requires consideration of the most ancient manuscript of his work, which has been preserved since 581 CE.[61] The Proto-John was a monk who lived in the region of Apamea in the northern part of Syria, and judging by the preserved manuscripts, his theological ideas were very

58 Cf. Jean D'Apamée, *Dialogue* 1, 1; Lavenant, *Dialogues*, 47.

59 All the argumentation about the identity of the three Johns of Apamea can be found in Irenée Hausherr, "Jean d'Apamée," *OCP* 14 (1948): 3-42; Lavenant, *Dialogues*, 17-19. In addition, Antoine Guillaumont also proposed the theory of the distinction of three persons with the same name. See Antoine Guillaumont, *Les 'Kephalaia Gnostica' d'Evagre le Pontique et l'Histoire de l'Origénisme chez les Grecs et chez les Syriens*, Patristica Sorbonensia 5 (Paris: Cerf, 1962), 196.317-319.335.

60 The nomenclatura of Proto-John, Deutero-John, and Trito-John is not used by the scholars cited in this work since it is a systematic classification established by the author of the present work.

61 Cf. Baumstark, *Geschichte*, 88-90; Ortíz de Urbina, *Patrologia syriaca*, 109.

much in vogue during the fifth and sixth centuries. He was an educated man who received a great deal of his formative experiences in Alexandria, as stated by Lavenant,[62] where he obtained a Hellenistic education including philosophy and logic, as well as biology and medicine, all of which held significant places in the Hellenistic instruction of the time. This pedagogical background helps explain the frequent use of the literary image of the embryo formed in the maternal womb as an analogy to illuminate the formation and development of the interior person who needs spiritual maturity to live in the invisible world. Such anthropological physiognomy helps John to perceive—by means of analogy—the spiritual physiognomy.[63]

The second John of Apamea was also from Syria, but the difference is that this Deutero-John professed a Gnostic pantheism and promoted the notions of Emanationism.[64] Most of the information about this "John" comes from Theodore Bar Koni, a Nestorian and Manichean heresiologist and Christian bishop from Mesopotamia who published his writings in Syriac, among which is found his Kṯāḇā 'eskoljōn, also known as the *Liber Scholiorum*, written around 790 CE. In this work, Bar Koni described the person in question—John the Solitary—as coming from Apamea in northern Syria.[65] This "Deutero-John" lived for a while in Alexandria, where he studied under the guidance of some magicians; when he returned to Apamea, he entered the monastery of Mar Samuel and Mar Shemun, also known as Deyr Ul Umur, which was founded in 397 CE.[66] In that region, he became notorious for his unorthodox theology. This heretical path created enemies for the Deutero-John of Apamea, among whom were Philoxenos of Mabbug, also known as Xenaias.[67] Regarding the figure of Philoxenos, David Michelson offers the following description of the charismatic leader:

> From his birth in Persia to his exile and death in Thrace (523), the life and work of the fifth-century bishop Philoxenos of Mabbug spanned remarkably varied geographic, political, and religious environments. Perhaps originally educated as a

---

62 Cf. Lavenant, *Dialogues*, 21.

63 Cf. Strothmann, *Johannes vom Apamea*, 65; Lavenant, *Dialogues*, 21-22, note 5.

64 Cf. Hausherr, *Jean d'Apamée*, 6-8; René Lavenant, "Le problème de Jean d'Apamée," *OCP* 46 (1980): 388-389; Id., *Dialogues*, 17.

65 Cf. Théodore Bar Koni, *Liber Scholiorum* (Corpus Scriptorum Christianorum Orientalium 66; Paris: Louvain, 1912), 331-333; L. J. R. Ort, *Mani: A Religio-historical Description of His Personality* (Leiden: E.J. Brill, 1967), 32-33.

66 The monastery in the seventh century began to be called the "Monastery of Mar Gabriel" after its bishop Mar Gabriel, who died in 668 CE.

67 The Syrian name of Philoxenus of Mabbug is Aksenāyâ Mabûḡāyâ, who died in approximately 523 CE.

dyophysite in Edessa, Philoxenos eventually became the miaphysite metropolitan of Mabbug (Hierapolis in Euphratensis). Active in the ecclesiastical politics of Antioch and Constantinople, Philoxenos also strategically used his location on the Euphrates to engage in missionary activity beyond the Roman Frontier both in Persarmenia and Arabia. Over the course of his ecclesiastical career, Philoxenos played the many roles of an experienced bishop: ascetic leader, theologian, exegete, patron of a revised Syriac New Testament, polemicist, and would-be imperial counselor. Philoxenos wrote prolifically leaving works in a variety of genres: polemics, Biblical commentary, homilies, doctrinal theology, letters, and ascetic paranaesis.[68]

The metropolitan of Mabbug has been listed traditionally under the heretical category of monophysite. This long-stereotyped view of Philoxenos has been challenged by Joseph Lebon,[69] André de Halleux,[70] and more recently by David Michelson, who proposed new approaches of scholarship that objectively uncover other aspects of the theology and thought of Philoxenos. This means that new scholarship needs to read the work of the theologian of Mabbug from viewpoints not limited by the monophysite controversy and the Christology of Chalcedon. There is no doubt that remains an unknown theologian who has been conceived as one of the most ardent monophysites and one of the beacons of Syriac literature between the ages of Ephrem and Jacob of Edessa.[71]

Philoxenos emerged as an ecclesiastical politician, a theologian, and a prolific author who tried to address a range of pressing issues among which, according to the information collected by Lavenant, included a heretical monk with the appellation of John the Egyptian. The appellative with the geographical determination is crucial because the different usage of the name in this case indicates to the reader that Philoxenos wanted to avoid any confusion of personality where the heretical monk could be erroneously identified with the spiritual master known as John of Apamea (Proto-John), who was certainly well known by Philoxenos.[72]

---

68 David Michelson, "Introduction to Hugoye 13: A Double Issue to Philoxenos of Mabbug," *Hugoye*: *Journal of Syriac Studies*, 13, no. 1 (2010): 3.

69 Cf. Joseph Lebon, *Le monophysisme sévérien* (Louvain: Impr. Orientaliste, 1909); Id., "La christologie du monophysisme syrien," in *Das Konzil von Chalkedon. Geschichte und Gegenwart*, eds. Aloys Grillmeier and Heinrich Bacht (Würzburg: Echter Verlag, [5]1979) I, 425-580.

70 Cf. André de Halleux, *Philoxène de Mabbog. Sa vie, ses écrits, sa théologie* (Louvain: Impr. Orientaliste, 1963).

71 Cf. Michelson, "Introduction to Hugoye 13," 3.

72 Cf. René Lavenant, "La Lettre à Patricius d'Édesse de Philoxéne de Mabboug," *PO* 30, no. 5 (1963): 848; Strothmann, *Johannes vom Apamea*, 81-90; Hausherr, *Jean d'Apamée*, 6.

The Third John of Apamea was from Mesopotamia, and he was also known as an unorthodox theologian who was condemned by Catholicos Timothy the First for his Messalian conceptions regarding prayer and sacraments in an eastern Syrian synod from 786–787 CE. In the same synod, John of Dalyatha, a Nestorian theologian, and an eastern Syrian monk named Joseph Hazzaya were also condemned for their Messalian tendencies that may have been influenced by the theological notions of the so-called John the Solitary (Trito-John).[73] Those referred to as Messalians (an Aramaic term used to indicate ones who pray) were also known by the Greek name of Euchites, which derives from the Greek verb προσεύχομαι (to pray), indicating their most important characteristic of life.

The Messalians were considered fanatics. Their movement originated in the region of Mesopotamia, Syria, and from the borders of Armenia around 360 CE. Their way of living Christianity spread rapidly in the fourth and fifth centuries throughout Syria and Asia Minor. Epiphanius of Salamis († 403 CE) mentions them in his *Panarion*[74] before the death of the Emperor Flavius Julius Valens († 378 CE). The Messalians were not organized as a structural movement; they were a group of monks, like that of the so-called Trito-John, or Christians attracted to the solitary or monastic life who had renounced their possessions and pleasures, living entirely upon alms. They were like nomads who did nothing except pray. Their attitude embodied a challenge to the ecclesiological dimension of the hierarchy and the liturgy of the church. They refused to accept the sacramental life of the Church and the liturgical devotions, fast days, and holy days established by the Church's offices and authorities. They believed that only by prayer and prayer alone could a person be saved and have a personal relationship with God. "According to them, baptism only effaces past sins; it does not prevent indwelling in every man, from the time of his birth, of an evil spirit with whom he has to struggle incessantly."[75] Their ascetic ways of practicing poverty, celibacy, self-denial, and fasting without the mediation of the sacramental life of

73 Cf. Lavenant, *Le problem*, 384-387; Strothmann, *Johannes vom Apamea*, 103-104; Isaac of Niniveh, *On Ascetical Life*, trans. Mary Hansbury (Crestwood, NY: St. Vladimir's Seminary Press, 1989), 18.20-21.

74 See the English translation of this work: Epiphanius of Salamis, *Panarion. Books II and II* (Sects 47-80; De Fide), trans. F. Williams (Leiden – New York – Köln: Brill, 1993). Daniel Caner affirms that Epiphanius' description of the Messalians is based upon hearsay, and the scrupulosity of the author compelled him to describe the Messalians by means of exaggerations and unfounded information. Later on, the so-called Messalian heresy received great attention among the ecclesiastical authorities, condemning it through several Synods. Cf. Daniel Caner, *Wandering, Begging Monks*, 86-91.

75 Louis Duchesne, *Early History of the Christian Church. From Its Foundation to the End of the Fifth Century* (London: John Murray Ltd., 1957), II, 461.

the church caused them to believe and proclaim that they were able to see God with their physical eyes. The Messalians, after causing so much controversy and alarm to the episcopate of the day, were finally anathematized by the Ecumenical Council of Ephesus (431 CE).[76]

---

76 The Definition of the Holy and Ecumenical Synod of Ephesus against the Impious Messalians who are also called Eucetae and Enthusiasts (found in Latin only. Labbe and Cossart, Concilia, Tom. III., col. 809): "When the most pious and religious bishops, Valerian and Amphilochius had come to us, they proposed that we should consider in common the case of the Messalians, that is the Euchetes or Enthusiasts, who were flourishing in Pamphylia, or by what other name this most contaminating heresy is called. And when we were considering the question, the most pious and religious bishop Valerian, presented to us a synodical schedule which had been drawn up concerning them in the great city of Constantinople, under Sisinnius of blessed memory: What we read therein was approved by all, as well composed and as a due presentation of the case. And it seemed good to us all, and to the most pious bishops Valerian and Amphilochius and to all the most pious bishops of the provinces of Pamphylia and Lycaonia, that all things contained in that Synodical chart should be confirmed and in no way rescinded; also that the action taken at Alexandria might also be made firm, so that all, those who throughout the whole province are of the Messalian or Enthusiastic heresy, or suspected of being tainted with that heresy, whether clerics or laymen, may come together; and if they shall anathematize in writing, according to the decrees pronounced in the aforesaid synod [their errors], if they are clergymen they may remain such; and if laymen they may be admitted to communion. But if they refuse to anathematize, if they were presbyters or deacons or in any other ecclesiastical grade, let them be cast out of the clergy and from their grade, and also from communion; if they be lay-men let them be anathematized.

Furthermore those convicted of this heresy are no more to be permitted to have the rule of our monasteries, lest tares be sown and increase. And we give command that the most pious bishops Valerian and Amphilochius, and the rest of the most reverend bishops of the whole province shall pay attention that this decree be carried into effect. In addition to this it seemed good that the filthy book of this heresy, which is called the Asceticon, should be anathematized, as composed by heretics, a copy of which the most religious and pious Valerian brought with him. Likewise anything savouring of their impiety which may be found among the people, let it be anathema. Moreover when they come together, let there be commended by them in writing such things as are useful and necessary for concord, and communion, and arrangement (dispositionem vel dispensationem). But should any question arise in connexion with the present business, and if it should prove to be difficult and ambiguous, what is not approved by the most pious bishops Valerian and Amphilochius, and the other bishops throughout the province, they ought to discuss all things by reference to what is written. And if the most pious bishops of the Lycians or of the Lycaonians shall have been passed over; nevertheless let not a Metropolitan be left out of whatever province he may be. And let these things be inserted in the Acts so that if any have need of them they would find how also to expound these things more diligently to others." See Council of Ephesus n. 240, in

Consequently, the so-called "Trito-John" is the most obscure figure among the three. The first two were very close in their chronological and geographical settings, rendering the confusion of identity between the two of them more understandable. That is why the appellative distinction made by Philoxenus of Mabbug is noteworthy. The third John, on the other hand, appeared in history in a posterior time, namely, in the seventh and eighth centuries, immersed in Nestorian and Messalian theological currents.

3.2. The Hypothesis of Two Different Persons

The foremost representative of the hypothesis of two different persons is Anton Baumstark, who believed in the existence of two people known as John of Apamea.[77] The first is John the Solitary from Orontes, who corresponds with the information given regarding Deutero-John, according to Hausherr and Lavenant. Baumstark used the information given by Bar Koni[78] to identify this John with the one who went to Alexandria to study medicine, logic, and rhetoric as the fundamentals of his intellectual formation. According to Baumstark, this John was influenced by the Neoplatonic and Pantheistic currents of his time, initiating from such an intellectual platform the construction of his Neoplatonic Christian speculations.[79]

The second John, from Mesopotamia, was involved in the Nestorian and Messalian theological conception, corresponding to the Trito-John of Hausherr and Lavenant. According to Baumstark, this John is the one who was condemned by Catholicos Timothy the First in 786–787 CE.[80] The John from Mesopotamia was a Nestorian theologian who, based on the theological notions of John of Dalyatha and Joseph Hazzaya, questioned the unity of the divinity and the humanity of Christ.[81] Their Christological argumentations contended with and denied the principal dogmatic belief of the one person of the Son—the in-

the *Nicene and Post-Nicene Fathers*, 2nd series, Vol XIV edition by H. R. Percival. It was digitized by Fordham University, Mediaeval Sourcebook: Council of Ephesus 431 (New York, 1996).

77 Cf. Baumstark, *Geschichte*, 166-167. 220-221.226.

78 Cf. Baumstark, *Geschichte*, 166. note 3.

79 Cf. Baumstark, *Geschichte*, 167.

80 Cf. Baumstark, *Geschichte*, 220-221.

81 Cf. Baumstark, *Geschichte*, 226.

carnated Logos—in whom there is a unity of two distinct natures, as previously established by the Council of Chalcedon (451 CE).[82]

3.3. The Hypothesis of One John of Apamea

Werner Strothmann argues that the idea that John of Apamea must be only one person. The three "Johns of Apamea" differentiated by Hausherr and Lavenant are just nuances or aspects of the same historical person who, in the present study, is called the Proto-John.[83]

Strothmann also used the information given by Bar Koni—as Hausherr and Baumstark did—to arrive at the conclusion of one historical person.[84] At this point, one might ask the following question: How can Strothmann explain the Nestorian and Pantheistic heretical notions in conjunction with the sound doctrine and spiritual teachings manifested in the writings of one single person through the history of circa 300 years?

After an exhaustive citation of John of Apamea's texts through a historical evolution of the quotations of his writings in other authors, Strothmann concludes that the wholesomeness and integrity of John's doctrine were corrupted over time between the second half of the fourth and the first half of the fifth century with the influence of Nestorian, Pantheistic, Gnostic, Messalian, and Neoplatonic notions that were never originally professed by the Syrian monk.[85]

4. Concluding Elucidations

The present work follows the line of reasoning presented by Hausherr and Lavenant. This research does not deny categorically the other theories proposed, but it is logically easier, according to the historical data of the witnesses reviewed, to acknowledge the existence of a group of theologian monks from the same geographical area who had the same name and, over a period of almost three centuries, presented in their writings diverse theological opinions that moved through a wide variety of theological positions. Some of the main obstacles to the acceptance of Strothmann's proposal turn out to be Philoxenos of

82 Cf. Heinrich J. D. Denzinger, *Enchiridion symbolorum, definitionum et declarationum de rebus fidei et morum. The Sources of Catholic Dogma*, trans. Roy J. Deferrari (St. Louis, MO: Herder, 1957), n. 148.

83 See the Vorwort of Strothmann, *Johannes vom Apamea*, i, 62-67.

84 For the development and argumentation of his theory, see Strothmann, *Johannes vom Apamea*, 81-115.

85 Cf. Strothmann, *Johannes* vom *Apamea*, 63-67.100-101.

Mabbug's affirmations, Palladius, Asemani, and Ebedjesu's information regarding the Syrian monks.

Philoxenos of Mabbug identified the existence of a certain John, an Egyptian heretical theologian, who cannot be mistaken for John of Apamea, an orthodox Syrian theologian. This historical fact indicates the possibility of erroneous misunderstandings of identity because of the commonality of appellatives. For this reason, Philoxenos was impelled to clarify the distinctiveness of the heretical monk by way of contrast, for the orthodox John of Apamea (Proto-John) was a well-known spiritual personage with a solid reputation. It would be difficult to explain this distinction if one were to assume that there was only one person whose notions and writings were manipulated or misunderstood.

The argumentation concerning multiple persons is corroborated by the writings of Palladius in his *Historia Lausiaca*. Palladius was born in Galatia circa 368 CE, dying probably before 431 CE. He was responsible for chronicling the life of John Chrysostom, the Bishop of Helenopolis, and compiling the meditations, stories, and reflections of the early Christian monks who lived in the Egyptian desert. The latter collection was written circa 419–420 CE at the request of Lausus, chamberlain at the court of the Byzantine Emperor Theodosius II, and this *opus* became known in the Christian tradition as the *Historia Lausiaca*.

Palladius had direct personal communications with a John of Lycopolis, also known as John of Egypt, the seer of Thebaid, a renowned ascetic who died in Thebaid, whose life he wrote about and from whom he attained precious information regarding various monks of Thebaid. The author of the *Historia Lausiaca* gives some of the first information about the writings and life of John the monk as the one who informed the emperor Theodosius concerning future things[86] and indicating that this John was the author of the letters to Eutropius and Eusebius and four discourses in the form of spiritual dialogues addressed to the same personages. The identification of John the Solitary of Apamea with John of Lycopolis according to this data is accepted by William Cureton and Sven Dedering, but Palladius gives in chapter 61 of his *Historia Lausiaca* an account of another "John" who was also a solitary monk of Thebaid and likewise had the qualification of a "seer." "This John is stated to have been the writer of letters and other works, whereas John of Lycopolis is not mentioned as an author."[87] The theological themes of the latter are the same subjects of the elucidations of the former. This John was contemporaneous with John of Lycopolis, but they cannot be the same person. The identification, assumed by Dedering

86 Cf. Cureton, *Corpus Ignatianum*, 351; Lightfoot, *Apostolic Fathers*, 153.

87 Lightfoot, *Apostolic Fathers*, 154.

based on the argument of possible persons from the same geographical region with the same theological themes and spirituality, becomes unsustainable. This "John", denoted in the present research as Proto-John, can be placed at the end of the fourth century or the beginning of the fifth, a spiritual father who had a common name and characteristics with other solitary monks who were contemporaries of Evagrius of Pontus and other monks of Thebaid and Apamea.

Giuseppe Simone Asemani, in his *Biblioteca Orientalis* volume I,[88] also corroborates the existence of other solitary monks who lived in different centuries with the same name of John the Solitary of Apamea. This identification is rejected by Cureton and Lightfoot, who see in Asemani's dating of this monk a lack of convincing arguments. Lightfoot, therefore, concludes regarding Asemani's hypothesis that "there is indeed, so far as I know, no reason why John, the Monk of Thebais should not be John of Apamea. There were many Syrians among the monks of the Egyptian desert. In this case, however, Asemani's date must be abandoned."[89]

The multiple persons theory also found a basis in the work of Ebedjesu, who in his *Syri Orientales* commentary[90] mentions two monks with the name of John. Concerning first of them, mentioned in chapter 39, the author gives no account of written work or theological production. The second, mentioned in chapter 47, is the one that Lightfoot would consider John of Apamea with the respective list of works already classified by Cureton and Wright. How are we to interpret this information from Ebedjesu? Historically, it means that there were two monks with the same name, or, as Lightfoot suggested, they are the same person mistakenly considered two distinct persons by Ebedjesu, which influenced Asemani's dating. The historical path that offers the possibility of different

88 Cf. Giuseppe Simone Asemani, *Bibliotheca Orientalis Clementino-Vaticana*: *In qua manuscriptos codices Syriacos, Arabicos, Persicos, Turcicos, Hebraicos, Samaritanos, Armenicos, Aethiopicos, Graecos, Aegyptiacos, Ibericos, et Malabaricos, jussu et munificentia Clementis XI Pontificis Maximi ex Oriente conquisitos, comparatos, et Bibliotecae Vaticanae addictos Recensuit, digessit, et genuina scripta a spuriis secrevit, addita singulorum auctorum vita, Joseph Simonius Assemanus, Syrus Maronita* (Rome, 1719-1728), I, 431, in *Apostolic Fathers*, 154.

89 Lightfoot, *Apostolic Fathers*, 154.

90 Cf. Georgius Ebedjesu Khayyath, *Syri Orientales, seu Chaldaei, Nestoriani et Romanorum Pontificum Primatus. Commentatio Historico-philologico-theologica*. Syriac Studies Library 105 (Piscataway, NJ: Gorgias Press 1870, 2011). See also Ebedjesu, "Metrical Catalogue of Syriac Writers," in *The Nestorians and Their Rituals*, ed. G. P. Badger (London: Joseph Masters and Co., 1852), II, 361-379. On page 368, Ebedjesu distinguished two different authors in his list of Christian fathers: "John wrote histories" and after listing seven names, he wrote, "John of Apamea wrote three books, and several epistles on the Spiritual Life, on the effects of Sin and on Perfection."

monks from the same or different periods continues to be, according to my position, the most acceptable solution to the problem of the authorship of these fourth to seventh century writings in Syriac since the writings of Palladius that present the same situation have not been considered a mistake.

If there were many Syrian monks in the Egyptian desert, which one was the author of the dialogues with Thomasios and the tractates regarding the soul published by Dedering, Strothman, Hausherr, and Lavenant? The fact that Palladius in his writings gives an account of two different persons with similar characteristics opens the door for us to accept as the most logical assumption the hypothesis of multiple persons. This balanced scholarly position resides in finding the most acceptable theory of explanation regarding the author of the works published in the twentieth century accredited to the so-called John of Apamea. Lightfoot, at the end of the nineteenth century, did not have the arguments and information of the research made by the German and French schools of the authors previously mentioned. Asemani's assumption, however, has great value for my present research because he already saw the possibility of a different Christian author who had the same characteristics as the one indicated by Palladius and Cureton but who lived in a different century. This hypothetical platform is the stepping-stone upon which the theories of three and two persons were elaborated.

Subsequently, if the multiple persons theory is taken as the most plausible proposal, it is possible to affirm that the second and sixth dialogues with Thomasios (alongside the other four mentioned by Lavenant) belong to the Proto-John of Apamea, a Syrian monk who was a master of spirituality and of whom Babai the Great said that he walked in the same path as Theodore of Mopsuestia and Evagrius Ponticus.[91] Therefore John the Solitary of Apamea can be taken into account even today as an ancient wealth of beneficial spiritual and theological notions that are ever relevant.

---

91 Cf. Hausherr, *Jean d'Apamée*, 182; Wilhelm Frankenberg, *Evagrius Ponticus. Abhandlungen der königlichen Gesellschaft der Wissenschaften zu Göttingen Philologisch-Historische Klasse*. Neue Folge 13, no. 2 (Berlin: Weidmannsche Buchhandlung, 1912), 135. See also a summary of the different theories about the identity of John of Apamea in Robert A. Kitchen, *In Search of Lost Apophthemata in John the Solitary of Apamea* (Regina, Saskatchewan: Knox-Metropolitan United Church, Independent Academia, 2012), 2-5.

Chapter II

John of Apamea's Significant Theological Notions

1. The Holy Scripture and John of Apamea

Evidence of a permanent exegetical and meditative interpretation of Scripture that a reader can perceive when reading the works of the Syrian monk is found in the spiritual affirmations, eschatological notions of the world to come, and hope in Christ, all of which are drawn from Scripture. The sacred text became the basic platform upon which John built his theological and spiritual architecture. The word of God became the *humus* of a spirituality where, with its roots set in the event of Christ, the kingdom of God is the ultimate goal. In this journey of the salutary economy, every person must walk through a path of purification in order to perceive the mysteries of God.

Biblical vocabulary and allusions to literary images of the Old and New Testament are embedded in the Hellenistic and anthropological philosophies of the author's milieu. He uses these words and references as intellectual instruments to present his Christian view of the total destiny of humanity that, as the history of the world continues to develop, will be fulfilled through the event of Christ, who provides proof for the final destiny of humanity, total communion with God according to his divine plan. The divine economy has been delineated through the experience of faith of the chosen people and the Christian community portrayed in Scripture, and therefore the sacred text provides for every age a non-exhaustive source of wisdom that illumines the path of everyone who assiduously reads it. For this reason, John calls it the "word of light."[1]

Continuous meditation on Scripture provided the author with the canvas to depict God's economy of salvation from the moment of creation up to the final and total fulfillment of human nature through the resurrection of Christ, who

---

1 Cf. Lavenant, *Dialogues*, 23.

gives to every person a foretaste of what will be in the world to come. As a product of his biblical reflections, John uses the synthetic expression: "economy of salvation" which summarizes the divine plan outlined in the biblical narratives. The Syriac term employed is *m^e^dabb^e^ronūto*[2] which is translated into Greek as οἰκονομία and into English as "economy." In modern terminology "economy" is related to financial transactions, including but not limited to investing funds, transactions, the stock market, etc. Therefore the modern semantic level of the term places it in a financial context.

According to the etymological Greek meaning, the word οἰκονομία can be found in the writings of Plato and Flavius Josephus, where it bears the meaning of the management of a household or the affairs implied in such activity. The term makes reference to the management, stewardship, oversight, and administration of a particular property. It also indicates the office of a manager.[3] The passage of Luke 16:2-4 presents this semantic field:

> He called him, and said to him, 'What is this that I hear about you? Give an accounting of your management (οἰκονομίας), for you can no longer be manager' (οἰκονομεῖν). The manager (ὁ οἰκονόμος) said within himself, 'What will I do, seeing that my lord is taking away the management position (οἰκονομίαν) from me? I don't have strength to dig. I am ashamed to beg. I know what I will do, so that when I am removed from management (οἰκονομίας), they may receive me into their houses.'

Therefore, the word οἰκονομία, applied to the field of theology, means the "plan of salvation," "order of salvation," or "the administration of salvation." In these translations, the theological meaning implies the general etymological significance. In 1Timothy 1:4 the term can be understood as godly instruction and God's work simultaneously, since it embodies the divine will of God for his people. The diversity in different renditions indicates the complex semantic levels of the term:

KJV: "Neither give heed to fables and endless genealogies, which minister questions, rather than godly edifying (οἰκονομίαν θεοῦ) which is in faith."[4]

NJB: "or to give attention to myths and unending genealogies; these things only foster doubts instead of furthering God's plan (οἰκονομίαν θεοῦ) which is founded on faith."[5]

---

2 Cf. Lavenant, *Dialogues*, 23.

3 Cf. BAGD, 559; Otto Michel, "οἰκονομίαν," *TDNT* V, 151-152.

4 King James 1611/1769, Blayney Edition 1988-1997.

5 New Jerusalem Bible, edited by Henry Wansbrough. Doubleday 1985.

NAS: "nor to pay attention to myths and endless genealogies, which give rise to mere speculation rather than *furthering* the administration of God (οἰκονομίαν θεοῦ) which is by faith."[6]

In a manner similar to the depth and richness of the meaning of the word economy (οἰκονομία) in a semantic context, as shown above, this term in the writings of the Syrian monk also entails different modalities in which the divine action of salvation is applied to human history presented from a communal and personal dimension. It is obvious to recognize that John takes inspiration from the Pauline theology. The apostle employs this terminology to describe the idea of the divine administration of human history, in which God is the most important character, controlling, changing, and catalyzing human events according to his design without eliminating human freedom and responsibility. Paul expresses the notion in a very personal manner in 1 Cor 9:16-17:

> For if I preach the Good News (εὐαγγελίζωμαι), I have nothing to boast about; for necessity is laid on me; but woe to me if I don't preach the Good News (εὐαγγελίζωμαι). For if I do this of my own will, I have a reward. But if not of my own will, I have a stewardship (οἰκονομίαν) entrusted to me.

The text indicates that the office of administrator or steward of the gospel (εὐαγγελίζωμαι) is a divine appointment, precisely given to a chosen person. The divine economy of salvation belongs to God, and he alone can appoint others to be administrators of the salvific actions in accord with his divine strategy. In Colossians 1:24-25, the apostle continues: "Now I rejoice in my sufferings for your sake, and fill up on my part that which is lacking of the afflictions of Christ in my flesh for his body's sake, which is the assembly, of which I was made a servant, according to the stewardship of God (οἰκονομίαν τοῦ θεοῦ) which was given me toward you, to fulfill the word of God." God himself provides the universal administration of humanity's salvation through the ministry or service of some persons chosen by him, among whom Paul considered himself a limited instrument in this universal project of God.[7]

Subsequently, the economy of salvation (οἰκονομία τοῦ θεοῦ) in John of Apamea's writings followed the Pauline line of thought. The Syrian theologian predominantly presents a dualistic conception of reality, namely the world from above and below, indicating that the divine economy includes all levels in the history of Salvation. His conception of creation and human history embodies a basic dualistic dimension in which the spiritual world and the celestial multitude of divine and angelic creatures will be indentified and perceived by humans be-

6 New American Standard Bible. Lockman Foundation 1977, 1995.

7 In this aspect of the Pauline vocabulary and theology see Gal 4:1-4; Eph 1:9-11; 3:2; 1 Tim 1:4.

ings without mediation in the world to come at the summit of the salutary history when humanity is resurrected and all human hope will be fulfilled in Christ.[8] In John's view, God created two worlds, the world of spiritual beings and the corporeal world, frequently denominated as physical or real world, within which humanity is immersed. But this notion is not derived exclusively from Platonic or Neoplatonic conceptions, as one can affirm simply after seeing its presentation above. These two worlds are not immiscible dimensions where one excludes the other; on the contrary, the spiritual realities exist, immersed and engaged with the corporeal and physical circumstantialities. In these intertwinings, the two dimensions relate to one another in the present world where humanity acts without seeing the dynamic action of the spiritual world interwoven in the historical progress of humanity.

The corporeity of humanity and the world presents itself as an instrument, albeit a challenging one, that the human person can use to ascend to the spiritual level of the mysteries of God. In other words, the present physical and bodily realm can be viewed as the training field through which one is able to obtain salvation.[9]

2. The Divine Pedagogy

Through the assiduous and attentive meditation on Scripture, John of Apamea was able to perceive a notion of the Divine Pedagogy that is patient and unwearied. Throughout the educational process, God instructs his people through the fluid course of historic events, in which Israel consistently manifests its unfaithfulness to his creator. The materiality and seductiveness of other gods and cultures caused Israel, who personifies Christian believers through history, to deviate from the bond of the covenant and love created by Yhwh who adopted Israel as his son.[10]

However, the material world wherein humanity interacts is not completely detrimental to the final destiny of the believer; it also serves as the amniotic sac in which the "interior person"[11] is forming like a fetus or an embryo in its mother's womb. When the moment of birth arrives, which occurs while the person is still living and acting in the material world, he or she begins the process of ma-

8 Cf. Lavenant, *Dialogues*, 23; Strothmann, *Johannes vom Apamea*, 25-26.

9 Cf. Lavenant, *Dialogues*, 24.102-104; Jean D'Apamée, *Dialogue* 5, 62-65. This notion is also manifested in Clement of Alexandria, *Paed.* 1,8,69; BAGD, 560.

10 Cf. Jer 3:19–20.

11 John of Apamea in his dialogues used the expression "interior man," embodying the totality of humanity or every person: male and female alike.

turity and learning that leads to complete independence, at which point the person is able to walk and interact effectively in the surrounding spiritual world.[12]

The anatomical image of the formation of an embryo, borrowed from his personal interest in medicine, helped John of Apamea to develop his delicate analogy of the spiritual person who needs the constant guidance and intervention of his or her divine pedagogue who is God himself. In the course of the complex apparatus of the physical world, God manifests himself continuously to the baptized—or the one who has faith—in the corporeal situations through many creative forms, persons, and events. In many creative and original ways, the spiritual pedagogue leads the person to recognize the realities of the invisible world. However, the functions or senses[13] of the spiritual person are numbed by the physicality of the body, which, hindering the perception of the spiritual senses, renders the spiritual person immersed in the material world incapable of clearly perceiving the spiritual reality.[14] The senses not being fully developed make someone incapable of perceiving with clarity the spiritual reality, because the spiritual person never had the opportunity to exercise this inner capacity of interacting with the spiritual realm. For example, in the material world babies' senses are not developed in the womb but they still can sense things. They start to respond to sound during the second trimester of their gestation and the exposure to sounds helps their ears grow accustomed to the relatively loud noises they hear after they are born. Thus the purpose of the divine pedagogical process is to make every person open to the knowledge of the mysteries of God given to us fully in the person of Christ through the economy of this world, mysteries that will be perfectly revealed in the spiritual state of the world to come. Then every person will exercise the superior senses and organs of the soul to their fullest capacity, becoming an integral and restored person in the transit from the visible worldly economy to the invisible economy.[15]

Seeing a direct connection between the notion of παιδεία manifested in the Alexandrian school through the writings and didactic conceptions of Clement, Origen, and Evragius with the notion of John of Apamea summarized above is possible. Since our working hypothesis postulates that the Proto-John, who is responsible of the six dialogues with Thomasios, was educated in the Alexandrian milieu, the Syrian monk most likely absorbed the integral philosophy of the Alexandrian spirit of education, which was not limited to the intellectual skills. The conception of education, pedagogy, included the art of thinking correctly

12 Cf. Jean D'Apamée, *Dialogue* 1, 9; Lavenant, *Dialogues*, 54-55.

13 The spiritual organs of perception are what is intended by the use of the expresion "spiritual sense".

14 Cf. Jean D'Apamée, *Dialogue* 1, 9-10; Lavenant, *Dialogues*, 54-55.

15 Cf. Jean D'Apamée, *Dialogue* 2, 19-20.60-62; Lavenant, *Dialogues*, 63-64.

with the tools of logic and philosophy, accompanied by psychological and spiritual formation through the Christian virtues. Therefore the pedagogy was at the same time a *psychagogy*. In other words, the concern of the Alexandrian school was for the soul to grow closer to God spiritually and intellectually.[16] Consequently for our ancient Christian authors, pedagogy was not a matter of the intellect alone, because the divine instruction is addressed to the heart and soul of the believer. This didactic methodology that aims at the totality of the person did not originate in the Alexandrian school. The care of the soul and the intellect within an educational system came from the Greeks or what we now refer to as ancient philosophy, as we can see in the writings of Plato and Aristotle.[17] Rather than simply being ideas and concepts that one memorized, philosophy at that time and place was a way of life, as Pierre Hadot puts it: "Thus as we have seen, philosophy in the Hellenistic and Greek period took on the form of a way of life, an art of living, and a way of being. This however, was nothing new; ancient philosophy had had this character at least as far as Socrates."[18] From this cultural platform the Christian writers built their pedagogy as a way of life that would characterize the future Christian thinkers and spiritual fathers.

The divine plan of education displayed in the salutary economy embodied a double dimension according to the Alexandrian Christian tradition that is also present in the pedagogical notions of John of Apamea. The first one is the divine providence that extends itself to each individual soul according to God's plan of redemption and salvation through his divine παιδεία. Second is the extension or manifestation of God's divine instruction in an inspired Christian teacher as an active participant of the salutary economy. A teacher is therefore a steward or dispenser (οἰκονόμος) of the divine plan, being an active instrument for the student's formation with charity and care for his or her soul and intellect.[19]

John of Apamea's six dialogues with Thomasios are an explicit expression of this double didactic dimension. On one hand, we see God as the divine pedagogue and architect of the universal plan of salvation; on the other hand, John conceived himself as a human instrument who participates harmoniously in the process of God's divine pedagogy and psychagogy. According to this line of thought, John the Solitary understood his position of a spiritual father as a steward (οἰκονόμος) who lead his disciples, more specifically Thomasios, to the

16 Cf. Judith L. Kovacs, "Divine Pedagogy and the Gnostic Teacher according to Clement of Alexandria," *JECS* 9, no. 1 (2001): 11.

17 Cf. Kovacs, "Divine Pedagogy," 12.

18 Pierre Hadot, *Philosophy as a way of life: spiritual exercises from Socrates to Foucault* (Oxford: Blackwell Publishing, 2003), 269.

19 Cf. Judith L. Kovacs, "Human participation in God's Plan: The Legacy of Clement of Alexandria," *JECS* 9, no. 1 (2001): 2.

knowledge of God and the heavenly realities through a virtuous life, experiencing in his own flesh the words of Paul: "So let a man think of us (Οὕτως ἡμᾶς λογιζέσθω) as Christ's servants (ὑπηρέτας Χριστοῦ) and stewards of God's mysteries (οἰκονόμους μυστηρίων θεοῦ)" (1Cor 4:1).

3. The Spiritual Physiognomy

Using his knowledge of anthropological Physiognomy and Scripture, John crafted his theological notion of the Spiritual Physiognomy, making him renowned among the Syrian writers. The spiritual doctrine of the Syrian author is centered in the marvelous gift of God to humanity, Jesus Christ. Implied most especially in this gift is the notion of the resurrection and eternal life that will be given to all humanity, according to God's wisdom. Thus faith, according to John, implies the belief in the resurrection of the dead and an endless life without sin to which every person is destined.[20] Christ gives this hope through baptism, which cleanses the person being baptized from sin and bestows on him or her the signs of the life to come. But before arriving at this future life in its fullness, the angelic state, a person must go through a process of purification. Rather than denying the earthly and material life, God's inclusion of this stage in his plans means that the current physical reality of a person's life becomes the particular starting point or the training field for achieving the state of perfection or *gmīrūtā*.[21]

There is, according to John's view, a tripartite order of the spiritual path of life which is based upon the tripartite dimension of a person. These three orders (taksīn) are the path of the body (somatic), the path of the soul (psychic/psychikos), and the path of the spirit (pneumatic), which also is called the pneumatic order. This notion is explicitly stated in John of Apamea's dialogue about the soul and the human passions:

> Il y a trois ordres d'hommes dénommés par l'Écriture: les somatiques, les psychiques, les pneumatiques... Est appelé somatique celui qui s'adonne aux convoitises de la nature du corps. Est psychique celui qui s'est élevé au-dessus des choses du corps et s'est approché de l'ordre de la nature de l'âme, c'est-à-dire qui combat contre la méchanceté de ses pensées, met un frein à son âme pour ne pas suivre ses instincts. Est spirituel celui qui est au-dessus des pensées corporelles et dont tout l'entendement se meut dans la sagesse qui est en Dieu.[22]

---

20 Cf. Jean D'Apamée, *Lettre* 1,82-84; Lavenant, *Dialogues*, 120-122; Jean D'Apamée, *Lettre* 2,92-93; Lavenant, *Dialogues*,128-129.

21 Cf. Lavenant, *Dialogues*, 28-29; Kitchen, *Apophthemagata*, 6.

22 Jean le Solitaire, *Dialogue sur l'âme et les passions des hommes*, ed. Hausherr, 13-14.

John of Apamea established this spiritual notion based upon the tripartite Pauline division of a person found in 1Thess 5:23: "May the God of peace himself make you perfectly holy and may you entirely, spirit (τὸ πνεῦμα), soul (ἡ ψυχὴ), and body (τὸ σῶμα), be preserved blameless for the coming of our Lord Jesus Christ."

The tripartite conception corresponds with the three stages of the spiritual path needed to achieve *gmīrūtā* (perfection). Thus in the spiritual journey a person may ascend or descend from one stage to another, as if one is going up and down a ladder. John's writings are not systematic theological tractates in the modern sense of the word. For that reason, his tripartite division does not indicate a clear or exact division between the three levels or paths. They are intertwined to the point that they can be experienced almost simultaneously, like someone walking concurrently on parallel paths.[23]

At this point of my exposition, a brief overview of the three orders according to the four dialogues regarding the soul and the human passions is fundamental.[24]

3.1. The Somatic Path

This order received the Syriac designation of *pagrānūtā*, which is the somatic state of the interior person. This state could easily be misunderstood by indentifying it with the lowest nature of the corporeal passions that cause a person to live an animalistic lifestyle without the direction or guidance of reason.[25] The *pagrānūtā* indicates the lowest level of spirituality in which the interior person is strictly attached to the corporeal senses and passions, not allowing the interior person to have true inner peace. This occurs because the interior person does not know another way of living than that of the physical body.[26] Therefore, the chief concern at this level is the fight against the passions, intended as the emotions and lustful desires contrary to the spirit,[27] in order to rise above them and enter into a superior spiritual state.

---

23 Cf. Kitchen, *Apophthemagata*, 14.

24 Cf. Johannes von Lycopolis, *Ein Dialog über die Seele und die Affekte des Menschen*, ed. et trans., Sven Dedering (Leipzig – Uppsala – Haag: Harrassowitz Verlag, 1936). See also Jean le Solitaire (Pseudo-Jean de Lycopolis), *Dialogue sur l'âme et les passions des homes. Traduit du syriaque sur l'edition de Sven Dedring*, ed. et trans., Irenée Hausherr, OCA 120 (Roma: Pontificio Institutum Orientalium Studiorum, 1939).

25 Cf. Brock, *The Syriac Fathers*, 79.

26 Cf. Paul Harb, "Doctrine spirituelle de Jean le Solitaire (Jean d'Apamée)," *PO* 2 (1971): 225-260 230.

27 BAGD, "πάθος," 602-603.

In Syriac two terms exist that can be used to signify the concept of passion. One is the word *zaw°o*, which simultaneously denotes the meanings of a movement (motion) and an impulse of the body and the intellect. The other term is the noun *ḥacho*, which signifies suffering.[28] According to this semantic determination, it is possible to distinguish two sets of passions, some that are compatible with the bodily level, and others that fit into the level of the soul. The passions of the body are "sleep, hunger, thirst, desire, intemperance."[29] The biological sexual instincts are the lowest manifestations of this kind, which can produce physical and moral suffering.[30]

While for the modern reader the psychological states might be more readily identified with the path of the passions of the soul, John also associates psychological states with the somatic path. These states can be the source of negative actions, depending on the context. It is important to understand that for John of Apamea some emotions or psychological states overlap the spheres of the *soma* and the *psychē*. John does not divide the boundaries of the three stages with the precision of a mathematical formula. The stages are fluid and extend themselves beyond their supposed limitations because the human person is an integral totality in whom all the anthropological dimensions are interconnected.

Some examples of these somatic states are recognized as "anger, zeal, jealousy, love of power, pride, boasting, lust."[31] The experience of "fear" can be qualified as one that also produces suffering. But conversely, it is possible to identify positive spiritual passions like "happiness, humility, and the love of God." These passions can facilitate a person's attaintment of a higher spiritual phase, allowing that person to advance further along the spiritual path.[32]

Each person who lives according to the path of the body struggles constantly against the passions, which become difficult obstacles in the process of ascending above oneself to the level of the invisible realities. The spiritual senses at the bodily stage are anesthetized, meaning that the interior person continues to relate to the physical world through the body, not perceiving the spiritual world properly. The progression to perfection therefore implies the surpassing of this level through the discipline, control, and purification of the body and mind, which requires continuous effort. This discipline also includes discerning be-

---

28 Cf. Lavenant, *Dialogues*, 40.

29 Johannes von Lycopolis, *Dialog* 2,43; Dedering, *Johannes von Lycopolis*, 5-6; Kitchen, *Apophthemagata*, 15.

30 Cf. Lavenant, *Dialogues*, 40.

31 Johannes von Lycopolis, *Dialog* 2,43; Dedering, *Johannes von Lycopolis*, 5-6.

32 Cf. Lavenant, *Dialogues*, 40.

tween the good and the bad passions of the body and soul, which in turn helps the person to move further along the spiritual pathway.[33]

3.2. The Path of the Soul

This spiritual order receives the denomination of *napšānūtā*. The stage of the soul, or psychē (ἡ ψυχὴ), can be located between the corporeal and the pneumatic level. The delimitation between these levels is fluid, namely, there is not a precise boundary between them. The person living in the *napšānūtā* struggles with the passions of corporeity and the passions of the soul concurrently.[34] The soul (ἡ ψυχὴ) is *per se* a spiritual entity, and while it has its roots in the corporeal body, it moves and acts in the realm of the invisible. For the modern reader, this stage would be equivalent to the intellect and the psychological functions of the mind. Through physical experiences, it is possible to have psychological experiences located in the psychosomatic range, where the two levels are conjointly experienced. In these cases, a person, elevated to a non-physical level where is possible to recognize the spiritual realm, is able to experience something in a non-corporeal dimension that cannot be measured by tangible tools.

How does one reach this point on the spiritual path? The question poses a real problem, since the Solitary does not give systematic answers. However, in his dialogues with Thomasios, the process of purification from evil things, despicable matters, and sinful thoughts is continually presented as the reliable path for a person to travel along in order to come to the level of being a person of the soul.[35]

3.3. The Pneumatic Path

This order, which is of the spirit, takes the Syrian name of *rūḥānūtā*. At this stage, the interior person experiences a harmonious unity of mind and spirit with the knowledge of the divine mysteries. Consequently, the interior person is able to perceive the invisible world immersed in the physical world through the senses of the spirit. The basic difference between the order of the soul (psychē) and of the pneumatic order resides in the special connection that the psychic order (*napšānūtā*) has with both the order of the spirit (*rūḥānūtā*) and the order of the body (*pagrānūtā*). The somatic order cannot exist apart from the corporeal reali-

33 Cf. Johannes von Lycopolis, *Dialog* 1,12; Dedering, *Johannes von Lycopolis*, 15-18; Kitchen, *Apophthemagata*, 15-16; Lavenant, *Dialogues*, 30-31.40.

34 Cf. Brock, *The Syriac Fathers*, 79.

35 Cf. Johannes von Lycopolis, *Dialog* 1,11–12.13; Dedering, *Johannes von Lycopolis*, 23-24; Kitchen, *Apophthemagata*, 16-17; Lavenant, *Dialogues*, 31.35.

ty of sensations and passions effected through physical experiences. The path of *pagrānūtā* serves as the bridge that connects the interior person with the order of the *psychē*. In the same way, the interior person cannot arrive at the pneumatic order without the experiences and perceptions developed in the stage of the *napšānūtā*. In this regard, John the Solitary affirms "since the soul's nature is spiritual—for the order of its nature is not the accomplishment of deeds, but the knowledge of the Spirit—if one elevates himself through his knowledge above the doing of the virtuous deeds, he no longer belongs to the order of the way of the soul, but to the spiritual order."[36]

This state of *rūḥānūtā* is characterized by *chafyûto*, which can be translated as "integrity." It implies the notion of purity, self-knowledge, and humility. In this stage the interior person is a spiritual essence capable of knowing the divine mysteries while being simultaneously united to a physical body in this world. "Purity of soul makes possible luminosity, or transparency of soul (shafyūt nafshā), which is a condition of receptivity to the light of the revelation of divine mysteries."[37] The spiritual state requires faith in Christ in order to undergo a process of total purification and awakening of the senses of the soul, so that the spiritual person can experience the invisible world and perceive the mysteries of the world to come.[38] This notion is correlated to the idea of interior transparency that belongs to the spiritual person who does not need any bodily contact or exterior manifestation to know the invisible world or the divine manifestations of God. The *rūḥānūtā* state cannot be perceived by a corporeal person, or even Satan and the demons. The spiritual transparency of the person in this state allows for the perception and experience of the mysteries of the invisible world through a life of total humility.[39]

3.4. Note of Conclusion

It is noteworthy to highlight that the tripartite anthropological dimension credited to John's theology appears exclusively in the four dialogues published under the title "Ein Dialog über die Seele und die Affekte des Menschen" by Sven Dedering, and its French translation under the title of "Dialogue sur l'âme et les passions des homes," edited by Irenée Hausherr. When we read other works attributed to John of Apamea, the tripartite anthropological division is not em-

36 Johannes von Lycopolis, *Dialog* 3,66; Dedering, *Johannes von Lycopolis*, 12-16; Kitchen, *Apophthemagata*, 18.

37 Cf. Brock, *The Syriac Fathers*, 79.

38 Cf. Jean D'Apamée, *Dialogue* 6,75-76; Lavenant, *Dialogues*, 42. 113-114.

39 Cf. Lavenant, *Dialogues*, 43-44.

ployed. Instead the reader discovers a dualistic anthropological conception prevalent throughout his theological elucidations.

John of Apamea's perception of humanity in relation to God is dynamic. The Syrian monk expresses his theological thoughts with flexibility, not following the patterns of classic systematic theology. However, in his dialogues, the solitary monk concentrates his anthropological and spiritual elucidations on two dimensions: the corporeal and the spiritual. For that reason, it will be helpful to have an overview of John of Apamea's second and sixth dialogue with Thomasios[40] to serve as proof and confirmation in order to demonstrate this dualistic notion that permeates most of the writings attributed to him.

40 See chapter III, sections 2,3, and 4.

Chapter III

John of Apamea and the Senses of the Soul

1. The Spiritual Senses

The expression "spiritual sense"[1] is *per se* a paradox. The spirit by its proper essence subsists independently from the body and the sensorial means that the person needs to communicate and interact with the surrounding world.

In antiquity, Platonic thought goes so far as to conceive of the soul as an entity that needs to liberate itself from the body and all corporeal functions in order to achieve its own perfection according to its nature, free from the trap of the corporeal human body. Therefore how is it possible to justify a paradox like "spiritual sense" in our study?

The notion of the spiritual senses in Christianity connects itself strictly to the event of the incarnation of the Logos: Καὶ ὁ λόγος σὰρξ ἐγένετο καὶ ἐσκήνωσεν ἐν ἡμῖν (Jn 1:14). Such an amazing event concretizes the notion that the invisibility of the spiritual world of God has become a sensory experience, emphasizing the bodily senses instead of rejecting them.

The Logos, through his incarnation, assumes a human nature, manifesting and revealing the mystery of God without the confusion or mixing of his two natures, divine and human. This means that the humanity of Christ is an instrument or channel of communication for the divine mystery; his flesh is not the divinity itself, since the human nature is not absorbed by the divine nature.[2]

1 The expression "spiritual sense," as it is used here, means the spiritual organs of perception.

2 The definition of the Council of Chalcedon (451 CE) confirms this statement: "Therefore, following the holy fathers, we all with one accord teach men to acknowledge one and the same Son, our Lord Jesus Christ, at once complete in Godhead and complete in manhood, truly God and truly man, consisting also of a reasonable soul and body; of one substance with the Father as regards his Godhead, and at the same time of one sub-

Thus the humanity assumed by the Logos becomes the means for the self-communication of God with the human race through the person of the Son. Jesus makes this statement explicit when he answers to Philip's question:

> Philip said to him, "Lord, show us the Father (δεῖξον[3] ἡμῖν τὸν πατέρα), and that will be enough for us". Jesus said to him, "Have I been with you such a long time, and do you not know me, Philip? He who has seen me has seen the Father (ὁ ἑωρακὼς ἐμὲ ἑώρακεν τὸν πατέρα). How do you say, 'Show us the Father?' (Δεῖξον ἡμῖν τὸν πατέρα;).[4]

The identification of the corporeal act of seeing (ὁ ἑωρακὼς) as leading to the perception of the mysterious reality of the Father through the visible human nature of the Logos exhibits the self-understanding within Jesus of his own identity, indicating the interconnectivity between the Trinitarian persons and the possibility of perceiving God through our human senses.

The anthropomorphic manifestations of Yhwh narrated in the sacred books of the first Testament reach their summit in the event of Christ. With the incarnation of the Logos in the person of Jesus, God, who is beyond any physicality, becomes accessible to humanity by means of the corporeal senses in a completely new (or radical) way. This physical experience of God does not exclude the realm of the spirit; quite the reverse is true: it assumes it. The relationship with God demands the totality of the human person, and experience of faith starts at the point of the physical sensibility that awakens the spirit through the faith in Christ: "Jesus said to him, 'Because you have seen me, you have believed (ὅτι ἑώρακάς με πεπίστευκας;). Blessed are those who have not seen, and have believed' (μακάριοι οἱ μὴ ἰδόντες καὶ πιστεύσαντες)" (John 20:29). Paul manifests

---

stance with us as regards his manhood; like us in all respects, apart from sin; as regards his Godhead, begotten of the Father before the ages, but yet as regards his manhood begotten, for us men and for our salvation, of Mary the Virgin, the God-bearer; one and the same Christ, Son, Lord, Only-begotten, recognized in two natures, without confusion, without change, without division, without separation; the distinction of natures being in no way annulled by the union, but rather the characteristics of each nature being preserved and coming together to form one person and subsistence, not as parted or separated into two persons, but one and the same Son and Only-begotten God the Word, Lord Jesus Christ; even as the prophets from earliest times spoke of him, and our Lord Jesus Christ himself taught us, and the creed of the fathers has handed down to us." Denzinger, *Enchiridion symbolorum,* n. 148.

3 δεῖξον is the imperative aorist active in the 2nd person singular of the verb δείκνυμι which can be translated as to show, point out, make known, (e.g. Matt 8:4; Lk 22:12; 1 Cor 12:31; Heb 8:5; Rev 1:1) explain, and prove (e.g. Matt 16:21). BAGD, "δείκνυμι," 172.

4 John 14:8-9.

the same idea according to his own experience of the kerygmatic proclamation in the apostolic era: "So faith comes by hearing (ἄρα ἡ πίστις ἐξ ἀκοῆς), and hearing by the word of Christ (ἡ δὲ ἀκοὴ διὰ ῥήματος Χριστοῦ)" (Rom 10:17).

This experience involving the senses opens the human soul to the reality of faith in the man and God Jesus Christ and becomes a spiritual perception. It is a perception that simultaneously includes the body and soul in order to elevate the person to the point where he or she can be considered a spiritual person. The physical and spiritual senses must interrelate to the degree that the latter aids the former in more readily perceiving the reality of the world, serving as a platform for the true mystical perception of the divine reality, as proposed by Corrigan: "the spiritual senses may well represent a more immediate and concrete way of seeing, a prelude to the greater immediacy of mystical seeing."[5] Here, all the functions of the person become spiritual, meaning that the person enters into the realm of the spirit to the point that he or she reasons and acts through the spiritual intellect and will. His or her spiritual sensibility unites the paradoxical extremes of the corporeal and spiritual means of perception in order to have a total and integrated experience of the visible and invisible world.[6] Therefore, the perception of the visible and invisible worlds are done through the spiritual heart, the spiritual imagination, and the spiritual senses. This phenomenon cannot be treated simply from a psychological point of view, because going beyond human psychology, it touches the realm of the spirit. Consequently, it must be studied from a theological point of view. For that reason, the aesthetic experience of a believer becomes spiritual.

Balthasar, in a very synthetic statement, establishes three *loci classici* from which the notions of the spiritual senses have been shaped through Christian history. These *loci classici* are the writings of three renowned figures: Origen, Bonaventure, and Ignatius of Loyola.[7]

One of the first explicit written manifestations of conception of the spiritual senses can be found in Origen, who developed it, in his own way, based on Platonic and Biblical analysis. His influence continued through the patristic period but the written manifestations of this notion are not as systematic and evident as in Origen's own writings. Through his allegorical application of exegesis, Origen perceived the spiritual meaning of the text that is rooted in its literal semantic manifestation. In this manner, he constructed his notion of spiritual aesthet-

5 Kevin Corrigan, *Evagrius and Gregory: Mind, Soul and Body in the 4th Century*. Ashgate Studies in Philosophy and Theology in Late Antiquity (Farnham, UK – Burlington, VT: Ashgate, 2009), 128

6 Cf. Hans Urs von Balthasar, *The Glory of the Lord. A theological Aesthetics* (San Francisco: Ignatius Press, 1982), I, 366-367.

7 Balthasar, *The Glory*, 367-368.372.373.

ics[8] taking into consideration pericopes like the text of Hebrews 5:14 "But solid food is for those who are full grown, who by reason of use have their senses (perceptions: τὰ αἰσθητήρια) trained by practice (γεγυμνασμένα) to discern good and evil."[9]

The Alexandrian author makes a clear distinction between the different semantic levels hidden in the Scripture and the capacity to read and discern them through the spiritual capacities of the intellect. The ability to understand the profound meanings of the Scripture is interconnected with the awakening and development of the spiritual perceptions. Regarding this notion, Origen establishes it in one of his meditations:

> Anyone who looks into this subject more deeply will say that there is, as the scripture calls it, a certain divine sense which only the man who is blessed finds on this earth. Thus Solomon says: 'Thou shalt find a divine sense.' there are many forms of this sense: sight which can see things superior to corporeal beings, the cherubim or seraphim being obvious instances, and a hearing which can receive impressions of sounds that have no objective existence in the air, and a taste which feeds on living bread that has come down from heaven and gives life to the world. So also there is a sense of smell which smells spiritual things, as Paul speaks of 'a sweet savour of Christ unto God', and a sense of touch in accordance with which John says that he has handled with his hands of the Word of life. The blessed prophets found this divine sense, and their vision and hearing were spiritual; in a similar way they tasted and smelt, so to speak, with a sense which was not sensible. And they touched the Word by faith so that an emanation came from him to them which healed them.[10]

There are therefore two sorts of senses: one kind is mortal, corporeal, and corruptible, and it is proper to the human bodily condition; the other kind is immortal and spiritual, for it belongs to the non-worldly nature of the human soul. These two sets of senses—meaning the organs of perception—are associated with one another, but the physicality of corporeal sensation does not allow the spiritual senses to be awakened in the interior person. Balthasar highlights a

---

8 In the writings of Euripides (V BCE), Epictetus (I-II CE), and Pre-Socratic Philosophers the term αἴσθησις signifies the perception by the senses. It indicates an experience and insight that denotes moral understanding. It also signifies intellectual perception and affection (love) for somebody. Origen applies this etymological value to the word "aesthetics" in order to express th spiritual perception of the divinity. See BAGD, "αἴσθησις," 25.

9 The text of Prov 2:5 and diverse passages of Song of Songs, among others, are also used by Origen because of their terminological connection with the notion of aesthetics (perception). Balthasar, *The Glory*, 368; Karl Rahner, "Le début d'une doctrine des cinq sens spirituels chez Origène," *RAM* 13 (1932): 113-145.

10 Origen, *C. Cels.* I:48, trans. Henry Chadwick (Cambridge – New York: Cambridge University Press, 1980), 44.

fundamental truth about the manner of interpreting Origen's notion of the spiritual senses. The reader must not take a rationalistic approach to the spiritual modalities of perception because the sacred text of Scripture refers to the divine revelation and manifestations of God in creation and human history. On the other hand, using the spiritual modalities of perception does not imply a simply mystical reading or interpretation of this phenomenon completely detached from an intellectual aspect. Consequently, reading and interpreting Scripture using Origen's notion of the spiritual senses requires an unbiased and balanced understanding of the notion of the five senses from a theological dimension.

Such a method of scriptural reading allows one to perceive and experience the presence of God present in the divine revelation of the Scripture as it was manifested to a human receptor capable of receiving it in and through his or her physical senses. These divine manifestation stimulate the spiritual sensibility of each person, drawing the person, ontologically capable of self-elevation, towards a theological view of reality and an elevation of the spiritual senses, to the point of experiencing the divine dimension of the Spirit in a way that truly feels real.

> Accordingly, the five individual sensory senses are but the fall and scattering into the material of an original and richly abundant capacity to perceive God and divine things. According to Origen, these divine things can never be reduced to a mystical unity without modes, but, rather, they possess a fullness and a glory that far transcend the lower fullness and glory, of which material multiplicity is only a distant reflection and likeness.[11]

The notion of the spiritual sensibility—or senses of the soul—continues to be alive through the middle ages and is present in the writings of the Syrian monks of the fourth, fifth, and sixth century, among whom is important to mention John of Apamea, who states in his second Dialogue with Thomasios the need for purification from the corporeal or terrestrial concerns in order to see the invisible realities through the superior senses of the soul. The Syrian Monk speaks explicitly of the analogy between the bodily senses and the senses of the soul, which make it possible for a corporeal person to perceive the invisible realities.[12] This notion of the spiritual senses also survived in the Christian Western Tradition, appearing in a more systematic manner in Bonaventure's *Itinerarium mentis in Deum.*[13] For Bonaventure, the spiritual senses are "the acts of the human intellect and will as they grasp God in contemplation; acts which have been restored (refecti), facilitated (expediti) and brought to perfection (perfecti) by the triple infused habitus of the 'virtues', the 'gifts of the Holy Spirit' and the 'beati-

11 Balthasar, *The Glory*, 369.

12 Cf. Jean D'Apamée, *Dialogue* 2,15-16 (SC 311: 59-61).

13 Cf. Balthasar, *The Glory*, 371-373.

tudes.'"[14] Reading these notions of Bonaventure, one can perceive that the division between the physical and spiritual senses is subtle, incorporating the virtues, intellect, will, and infused gifts. The enumeration of these different dimensions of a person indicates a complete and integral anthropological notion, where every person in his or her ontological being has the capacity to experience, bodily and spiritually, the Word of God in the divine economy.[15]

In the sixteenth century, Ignatius of Loyola in his *Exercitia spiritualia*[16] revives the notions of sensory experience in the field of spirituality. The person must use the bodily capacities to awaken or stimulate emotions and experiences that go beyond the corporeal sensations, helping the retreatant—the believer—to enter into the spiritual experience of faith in Christ's mystery. In the first prelude of the first exercise, Ignatius sets as a principle that one should start out on a spiritual path that does not deny the humanity or corporeity of the person. Thus the *first prelude* turns out to be the composition of the situation, meaning that the person should recreate the scene portrayed in the passage of Scripture and see the specific setting of the meditated event as forming an integral part of it. In this way, the retreatant becomes part of the biblical text or meditation, experiencing it in the totality of his or her being. Ignatius affirms:

> Here it is to be noted that, in a visible contemplation or meditation—as, for instance, when one contemplates Christ our Lord, Who is visible—the composition will be to see with the sight of the imagination the corporeal place where the thing is found which I want to contemplate. I say the corporeal place, as for instance, a Temple or Mountain where Jesus Christ or Our Lady is found, according to what I want to contemplate. In an invisible contemplation or meditation—as here on the Sins—the composition will be to see with the sight of the imagination and consider that my soul is imprisoned in this corruptible body, and all the compound in this valley, as exiled among brute beasts: I say all the compound of soul and body.[17]

The founder of the Jesuits saw in the use of the corporeal senses an intrinsic correlation with the soul, to the point that the usage of the corporeal senses is needed in order to have a spiritual experience. During the first week, the fifth exercise consists in the meditation of hell, and the way one can experience it is through the use of the senses in order to feel personally its reality. Having the understanding of its ugliness, which stands in sharp contrast with the wholeness of the divine economy in Christ, the retreatant will have the will to do every-

14 Balthasar, *The Glory*, 372.

15 Cf. Balthasar, *The Glory*, 372-373.

16 The First Edition of the *Exercitia spiritualia* was done by Antonio Bladio in Rome, 1548.

17 Ignatius of Loyola, *Spiritual Exercises*, trans. Elder Mullan (New York: Kennedy and Sons, 1914) 31.

thing it takes to avoid it. The two preludes to this step testify to the composition of place by the imagination with the full inclusion (or application) of all the corporeal senses.

> First Prelude. The first Prelude is the composition, which is here to see with the sight of the imagination the length, breadth and depth of Hell. Second Prelude. The second, to ask for what I want: it will be here to ask for interior sense of the pain which the damned suffer, in order that, if, through my faults, I should forget the love of the Eternal Lord, at least the fear of the pains may help me not to come into sin.[18]

Then Ignatius states an illuminating point for the usage in the meditation of every single physical sense, namely, that each must be helped by the intellect and the imagination, making the total experience more effective because it involves the body, intellect, and spirit:

> First Point. The first Point will be to see with the sight of the imagination the great fires, and the souls as in bodies of fire. Second Point. The second, to hear with the ears wailings, howlings, cries, blasphemies against Christ our Lord and against all His Saints. Third Point. The third, to smell with the smell smoke, sulphur, dregs and putrid things. Fourth Point. The fourth, to taste with the taste bitter things, like tears, sadness and the worm of conscience. Fifth Point. The fifth, to touch with the touch; that is to say, how the fires touch and burn the souls.[19]

This methodology is applied to every step of the exercise, starting systematically with the composition of the place or the life setting of the mystery on which one is supposed to meditate. For instance, during the second week the retreatant must meditate the mystery of the nativity, but as a prelude to it, that person must mentally compose the setting in order to experience the mystery in a personal and intimate manner:

> Second Prelude. The second, a composition, seeing the place. It will be here to see with the sight of the imagination the road from Nazareth to Bethlehem; considering the length and the breadth, and whether such road is level or through valleys or over hills; likewise looking at the place or cave of the Nativity, how large, how small, how low, how high, and how it was prepared... First Point. The first Point is to see the persons; that is, to see Our Lady and Joseph and the maid, and, after His Birth, the Child Jesus, I making myself a poor creature and a wretch of an unworthy slave, looking at them and serving them in their needs, with all possible respect and reverence, as if I found myself present; and then to reflect on myself in order to draw some profit.[20]

18 Ignatius of Loyola, *Spiritual Exercises*, 36.

19 Ibidem.

20 Ignatius of Loyola, *Spiritual Exercises*, 45.

In this kind of exercise the retreatant must be attuned to the situation selected, concentrating through his or her mental strength on the object of meditation which is the mystery of Christ. In doing so, the person includes the sensory dimension that then stimulates the spiritual sensibility, with the result that the person reaches a new dimension where God can communicate himself directly to the retreatant through a spiritual experience.[21]

The conception of the senses of the soul exhibits the analogy existing between the corporeal senses and their respective spiritual counterparts. As physical beings, humans have the sensory organs necessary to register impressions and experiences of the physical world by seeing, touching, smelling, tasting, and hearing. Analogously, the spiritual organs of perception, so to speak, allow the person to experience the divine or supernatural realities immersed in the existential chain of events, giving the person a generic divine sense (*theias aisthēseos*) of the presence and action of God.[22]

When applying the criteria of the spiritual senses as hermeneutical reading for Mark's Gospel, we must understand that the author of the Markan Gospel did not have in mind the notion of the five spiritual senses, in the same way as it was developed by Origen and the subsequent tradition. The Gospel therefore is not a systematic dissertation of spiritual perception. However, when the text is considered from this perspective, it shows that the author knew or conceived of a certain distinction between seeing physically and seeing spiritually, which makes it possible to affirm that the intuition or the perception of two realities, the physical and the supernatural, subsists in an interconnected manner in Mark's narrative. Of course, this notion is not expressed in the words of a systematic theological treatise, for the author describes the event of Christ according to the language proper to the kerygmatic genre, which narrates the deed and teachings of the son of God.

Applying to Scripture the notion of the spiritual senses helps the reader to discover different semantic levels in the narrative. Among the intricate and profound levels of communication implied in the sacred text, the reader can recognize and identify the diverse portraits of seeing in Jesus, the demons, and the women. These portraits of seeing induce the reader to conclude that their way of perceiving the realities or events in the account does not stop at the physical phenomenon but goes on to notice the divine immersed and hidden in the particular circumstances. Thus, the manner in which Jesus sees according to the physical and spiritual eyes occurs concurrently. His sensory organ of sight is in com-

21 Cf. Balthasar, *The Glory*, 373-376.

22 Cf. Patricia Cox Miller, *Dreams in Late Antiquity: Studies in the Imagination of a Culture* (Princeton, NJ: Princeton University Press, 1994), 94. Also see Origen, *C. Cels.* I:48 (Chadwick, 43-46).

plete harmony with the divine nature of his soul, allowing him to perceive every physical reality simultaneously at a spiritual level, which renders him capable of comprehending and scrutinizing the totality of each person. Therefore, the Markan portrayal of the seeing of Jesus corresponds to the seeing of God: total, penetrating, personal, and effective. The demons, being supernatural entities, are able to perceive the realities appertaining to their realm, and when they possess a person, the demoniac's sensory organ of sight synchronizes with the analogous spiritual and physical sense of the possessed person in order to identify and recognize instantly the supernatural identity of Christ. The women represent the believer who, in the middle of the confusion caused by the tragedy of losing a loved one, continues to contemplate the event of the death of the Lord.

John of Apamea's spirituality and theological notions regarding the spiritual senses are expressed in a manner that can be called a narrative of discursive theology, which is a different theological style and method from the ones developed by Origen, Bonaventure, and Ignatius. John's second dialogue with Thomasios is constructed upon the basis of the superior senses of the soul, the spiritual world, and the new world of the eschatological times, all of which are in contrast or in relationship with the notion of the corporeal senses, the material world, and its imperfections, which do not allow a person to perceive the beauty of the supernatural realities already manifested in the present world. This line of thought is also present in the sixth dialogue with Thomasios, but the theme is not as central as it is in the second dialogue. Nevertheless the same theological notion can be read in the latter text of our author, which is connected with other spiritual matters.

The following sections of this chapter expound the content of the second and sixth dialogue of John of Apamea with Thomasios. It is crucially important at this point to highlight that the content presented does not pretend to be a literal translation of the dialogues but rather a summary of their content, for there is not a critical or official translation of these two dialogues in English.[23]

2. The Content of the Second Dialogue with Thomasios (Syr. 2,13-21)

The second dialogue with Thomasios, which is attributed to John of Apamea (or Prot-John), was composed in the early stages of the fifth century. It is a result of the synthesis of the Greek and Syrian traditions regarding the knowledge of the

23 The information presented is based upon the critical edition of Sources Chrétiennes by René Lavenant. See René Lavenant, ed. et trans., *Jean D'Apamée. Dialogues et Traités. Introduction, traduction et notes*, SC 311 (Paris: Les Éditions du Cerf 1984).

divine. The second dialogue is a conversation with Thomasios, who, as recounted in the first Dialogue,[24] received an excellent Greek education, but being a man with a strong faith in Christ, he adopted the Solitary Syrian monk as his spiritual master in order to learn more about the Christian spirituality of the monastic and solitary life. John took this opportunity to teach Thomasios about the knowledge of God and the hope of the new world to come in eschatological times. In doing so, John offers a different perspective from the Greek epistemological tradition in which one's physical experience and observation of facts leads to certain conclusions about reality and truth.

During this second dialogue, Thomasios asks three questions, which function as the stepping ground for his master to explain the Christian tradition of the spiritual realities already developed by Origen in his meditations and studies regarding the Scripture.[25]

The first question considers the lack of agreement among the immense variety of knowledge and sciences. If they are looking for the truth in their respective fields, then why do they contradict each other, not retaining anything certain in mutual agreement?

To solve the problem regarding the diversity and multiplicity of sciences and knowledge, John shows how the mystery of Truth is intrinsically related to the nature of God. The multiple fields of knowledge therefore manifest the richness of God and the impossibility for any creature to comprehend fully his mystery and nature. Being by nature without a body, God manifests himself in multiple ways in the corporeal world under visible forms so that he can be known by creatures. Furthermore, if God was by his essence visible, it would be impossible for him to manifest himself in a plurality of forms, and any knowledge of him inherently limited, as he would be an object of study like any other in the realm of our experience, such as a dog or a tree. But since he is invisible, he can reveal himself in diverse forms, and in this way, our potential for knowledge of God is limitless. Since God wants to be known by his creatures, especially human beings, God makes himself known to humankind through the elements of this world, motivating all the sciences and tractates of the present era speak of God.[26]

John continues explaining that God will be able to be perceived in the same manner that a person can perceive visible realities like fire, air, and light, thanks to a new way of seeing by pure grace in the world to come. At that time all lan-

---

24 Cf. Jean D'Apamée, *Dialogue* 1,1; Lavenant, *Dialogues*, 47.

25 Cf. Origen, *C. Cels.* I:48, ed. et trans., Henry Chadwick (New York: Cambridge University Press, 1980) 44.

26 Cf. Jean D'Apamée, *Dialogue* 2,13-14; Lavenant, *Dialogues*, 58-59.

guages, explanations, and mere humanly knowledge will cease,[27] since the knowledge of God will be uncovered by himself, being explicitly present and accessible. But at the same time, it will be impossible for a person to comprenhend, interact with, and be formed by the immediacy of knowing God in the world to come without the interior senses proper to this life.[28]

Following the previous conclusion of his master the second question of Thomasios is: "Why is it that we cannot reflect on or understand anything?" This query opens the door for John to enlighten Thomasios about the notion of the invisible realities present in the corporeal human world. Inserted or hidden in the concrete and corporeal person, one can find the invisible reality of the soul, which is able to perceive and know the invisible realities of the spiritual domain. The problem of the corporeity in which the soul is embodied consists in the obstacle of the sensory organs that, not being properly exercised, do not allow the soul to recognize the hidden truth of the spiritual world immersed in the physical world. The body, perceiving only what is proper to its nature, becomes an impediment to the soul, for the spiritual senses are obstructed by the physical condition of the body, which does not allow the recognition and perception of what is spiritual. In order to demonstrate this aspect, John uses the analogical example of the lame man whose feet render him incapable of marching unless they are healed, or a blind man whose eyes cannot see unless they are cured and opened to the world, or a paralyzed tongue unable to utter a word until it is made well. Likewise the invisible spiritual senses, when they are impeded or damaged, cannot perform rightly. Evil habits, perverse thoughts, weaknesses, and the limitations of terrestrial things make the spiritual senses ill and incompetent in the exercise of their functions, which have as their ultimate goal the knowledge of God's mysteries.[29] The spiritual organs of perception become numb and atrophic when they are not in use, but when exercised by the soul, they are able to comprehend and perceive the spiritual sphere immersed in the present world, giving the person true knowledge and understanding.

When humankind cannot find fulfillment by spiritual knowledge, it is because, weakness of the human person that impedes the perception of the spiritual richness present and not some weakness or unwillingness on God's part. Continuing to use analogies to elucidate spiritual mysteries, John returns to the exam-

27 1 Cor 13:8: "Love never ends. But if there are prophecies, they will be set aside; if there are tongues, they will cease; if there is knowledge, it will be set aside". John at this point of his dialogue, quotes the second part of the verse: "if there are tongues, they will cease; if there is knowledge, it will be set aside" (8b). See Jean D'Apamée, *Dialogue* 2,15; Lavenant, *Dialogues*, 59.

28 Cf. Jean D'Apamée, *Dialogue* 2,15; Lavenant, *Dialogues*, 59-60.

29 Cf. Jean D'Apamée, *Dialogue* 2,15-16; Lavenant, *Dialogues*, 60-61.

ple of the eyes of a blind man who is not able to see the light in front of him, for when light shines forth before the blind man, his privation of vision hinders him from admiring and seeing what is in his presence. Like healthy eyes that allow a person to see, the invisible senses of the soul allow the person to perceive and understand the spiritual realm around him or her, but if they are not open to the reality of God, wisdom and knowledge of him cannot be acquired in this world. The therapy suggested by John is the purification of corporeal thoughts and worries in order to ascend to spiritual concerns. Regarding this, John states: "if we purify ourselves of wickedness, then we will come to see invisible realities. But there is no point, while we are still blind, in asking why it is we cannot see the light, no point in stuffing our ears and then asking why it is we cannot hear anything."[30] The same could be said about the soul who, being a prisoner of the corporeal world, cannot sense the invisible mystery surrounding it.

John also affirms that these ubiquitous obstacles can be overcome in the present life through the healing of the spiritual senses, which can be accomplished in the process of searching for the spiritual reality of God and his manifestations in this world, causing the human soul to ascend to the elevated grace of the invisible realities. The complete perception of the spiritual sphere will be achieved in the new world when the spiritual senses are totally open and healed to comprehend the divine wisdom.[31]

Thomasios' third question focuses on what the sign will be that humankind will be better than what they are in the present time, and when will that sign occur. At this point, John applies the argumentative demonstration of Paul's teaching, using Hebrews to highlight the faith of the forefathers, beginning with the Patriarchs, and emphasizing progressively the examples of faith that surpass the Law and please God. The total faith of mankind thus makes possible the accomplishment of a glorious economy of salvation that elevates each person to a state of perfection: "God had foreseen (προβλεψαμένου)[32] something better for us, so that without us they should not be made perfect (should not be fulfilled: τελειωθῶσιν)" (Hebrews 11:40).[33] For John, this period of perfection that, ac-

30 John Anthony McGuckin, ed., *The Book of Mystical Chapters. Meditations on the Soul's Ascent from the Desert Fathers and other early Christian Contemplatives* (Boston, MA / London, UK: Shambhala, 2003) 21. McGukin in his book only presents this paragraph translated from the second dialogue. See also Jean D'Apamée, *Dialogue* 2,17; Lavenant, *Dialogues*, 60.

31 Cf. Jean D'Apamée, *Dialogue* 2,17-18; Lavenant, *Dialogues*, 61-62.

32 προβλεψαμένου is the participle aorist of the verb προβλέπω, a derivative of βλέπω. It means to foresee or see beforehand, looking forward, provide or select. Cf. BAGD, "προβλέπω," 703.

33 Jean D'Apamée, *Dialogue* 2,19; Lavenant, *Dialogues*, 63.

cording to God's economy of salvation, will be completed in the world to come, has already begun in the corporeal world. This point demonstrates the paradoxical relationship between the spiritual and the corporeal anthropological dimension in John's theological notions. Humanity's corporeity functions as the obstacle that keeps the spiritual senses numb and prevents them from functioning, but at the same time, through the connection existing between the bodily and spiritual senses, the first step in stimulating the organs of the soul is through the purification of the corporeal ones so that the senses of the interior person can be utilized to their fullest capacity and according to their nature.

According to the images employed by the Syrian spiritual father, every person is present in the maternal bosom without perfect definition of his or her bodily parts, and by the grace of God, the time arrives when the person is mature enough to emerge into the world in order to continue living and developing. In the same way in which every person in this corporeal world is physically being formed, growing, and maturing, his or her spiritual senses are also developing, but they are not capable of functioning effectively until the person arrives, by the grace of the salutary economy, at the spiritual state where he or she will be able to apply the superior senses of the soul efficiently in order to perceive and comprehend the spiritual world.[34]

This invisible economy of God, proper to the imperceptible world, became part of the visible world, when the economy of salvation became part of humanity through the incarnation of the Logos. Through the person of Jesus every infirmity, deformation or unwholesomeness of the spiritual senses disappears, restoring the human person to the original state of beauty before God and giving humanity the possibility of enjoying the true happiness that comes from contemplation of spiritual mysteries. Without the healing of the spiritual senses, it would be impossible for any person to immerse themselves in the glory of the new world.[35]

John finishes his dialogue with Thomasios with the idea that the corporeal reality of a person becomes a handicap for the superior senses of the soul. But it is necessary to know corruption, because such knowledge facilitates an awareness of immortality and the true spiritual reality of the mysteries of God: "It is sown in dishonor; it is raised in glory. It is sown in weakness; it is raised in power" (1Cor 15:43).[36]

34 Cf. Jean D'Apamée, *Dialogue* 2,18-19; Lavenant, *Dialogues*, 62-63.

35 Cf. Jean D'Apamée, *Dialogue* 2,20; Lavenant, *Dialogues*, 64.

36 Jean D'Apamée, *Dialogue* 2,21; Lavenant, *Dialogues*, 65.

3. The Content of the Sixth Dialogue with Thomasios (Syr. 6,70-81)

Nine interventions of Thomasios assist the conversation with John the Solitary in this dialogue, regarding the revelations and visions of the divine economy in this world and the revelation of the economy of the world to come, intertwined with other subjects of diverse degrees of importance.

In the present study, the essential notion is related to the senses of the soul. In this regard the sixth dialogue follows the same line of theological thought of the second.

Thomasios' intervention about the human appearance of an angel becomes the stepping stone for John to talk about the invisible senses and the corporeal senses. John's response begins with the notion of a corporeal mass placed between the soul and God, which is an obstacle for the soul's clear vision and understanding of the supernatural; for this reason the perceptible human appearance of the angel becomes the bridge that allows corporeal human perception to catch a glimpse of another reality, the domain of the spirit, proper to the angels and God. The soul's senses are anesthetized by corporeity, and in order to awake them, it is indispensable that the divine makes itself known to humanity by means of physical manifestations. But the bodies of the world to come will be superior to corporeal entities since they will have been formed out of a spiritual substance. Consequently, the intermediation of physical appearances that allow persons to recognize and comprehend the spiritual mysteries will not be required. As every person can see the visible things of this world, in the world to come, everyone will be able to see the presently imperceptible qualities and beings without any need of intermediaries.

At the present moment, everything noticeable by the eyes of the body is corporeal and verifiable, and because God can reveal himself through physical bodies, the capacity to know the divine mysteries is part of the inherit essence of the human soul. Consequently, the human spirit has the *capax* of knowing spiritually but always through the grace of the revelation that is given. This divine economy has been present throughout human history, for God has been manifesting himself to humanity, sometimes assuming human or corporeal forms, in order to aid his human receptors in understanding him and his divine actions.[37] For that reason, the economy developed in the physical world consists of corporeal promises, which is the approach God takes to manifest himself during the historical period called the somatic era, which is the age before Christ.

37 Cf. Jean D'Apamée, *Dialogue* 6,71; Lavenant, *Dialogues*, 112.

With the event of the incarnation, the salutary economy reaches a higher level in the knowledge of God's mystery because the Trinitarian God manifests himself in a new manner to humanity. The Logos, through his incarnation, elevates the human condition to a supernatural dimension. Therefore, the divine kenosis of the Logos reveals the true finality of the human condition which is to be in a harmonious relationship with God. Through the two natures, divine and human, of the second person of the Trinity the divine dimension is able to be immediately present to the human condition, because the event of Christ, beginning with his incarnation and concluding with his resurrection, marks the beginning of a new period in the economy of salvation, which is called, by John of Apamea, the pneumatic era.

When the human soul is able to surpass the limits of the body, it can contemplate the unseen realities of God, in this way existing in a state of intimacy with God, which entails a laborious path of self-purification. When the soul is able to reach this point in the spiritual life, it will no longer need the physical senses to perceive and understand divine manifestations, but simply with the senses of the soul, a person will begin to comprehend the divine mysteries manifested in the present world that conjointly contain the inscrutable mysteries of the world to come. John continues his argumentation based upon his reflection on the letter of Paul to the Ephesians, stating that the revelation of the mysteries of the new economy will be manifested to the interior man, meaning the human soul, indicating the superiority of such an economy in relation to the previous one manifested through the prophets: "that the God of our Lord Jesus Christ, the Father of glory, may give you a spirit of wisdom and revelation resulting in knowledge of him" (Eph 1:17). This revelation mentioned by Paul is different from the one announced by the prophets, who did not have direct and personal encounter with Christ and died hoping for the coming of the Messiah. For this reason, Paul continues in his letter saying: "May the eyes of your hearts be enlightened, that you may know what is the hope that belongs to his call, what are the riches of glory in his inheritance among the holy ones" (Eph 1:18), indicating that with this new manifestation started with Christ, God reveals himself to the interior man.[38]

In John's answer to Thomasios' question regarding the nature of the angels, demons, and human soul, the Syrian spiritual master, quoting Ephesians 1:18, Deuteronomy 32:39, and Psalm 46:11 affirms that a person cannot see God with corporeal eyes. Only the seeing of the interior person can obtain an understand-

38 Cf. Jean D'Apamée, *Dialogue* 6,76; Lavenant, *Dialogues*, 114. The expressions "interior man" or "exterior man" are equivalent in John of Apamea's dialogues to the "human soul" and to "human corporeity."

ing of God. Therefore the seeing of the spiritual nature experiences and grows in the knowledge of God according to its capacity, since the knowledge of God attained by each spiritual nature is not equal. For this reason, the human soul cannot see and know as the angels do. The demons likewise cannot see and know as the angels do either, since the evil spirits cannot tolerate the *grandeur* of God.[39]

John concludes his dialogue with Thomasios by emphasizing that the true revelations of the new life are able to be understood and perceived by the human soul only when the person is able to rise above the tumult of his or her own thoughts, which are spiritual obstacles. In this part of his conversation with Thomasios, the Solitary monk centers his attention on spiritual perception and understanding, alluding to hearing because even without the ears, the human soul can understand divine revelations. This communication is possible because God can speak or communicate to a person without the sound of his voice, establishing a new and direct mode of communicating with the person in the undetectable and spiritual intimacy between the interior person and God. Hence every person is called to keep this hope in mind and not to allow human thinking to keep each of us trapped in this world.[40]

4. Corollary

The reader can perceive in John's second and sixth dialogue that the monk does not structure and develop his dialogues as systematic theological tractates of the spiritual senses. The style of the Syrian author consists in expounding his dialogues as a fluid theological conversation with his disciple, in which the notion of the invisible senses of the soul are utilized in order to discover the supernatural reality of God already manifested in this corporeal world. In these two dialogues, the Syrian monk never makes use of the anthropological tripartite notion for the spiritual development of the person. Similarly, he never mentions the three paths (somatic, psychic, and pneumatic) when answering any question of Thomasios. On the other hand, John bases all his responses and reflections upon the dualistic notion of body and soul that corresponds to the somatic and pneumatic orders (taksīn). Furthermore, the examples related to the corporeal and spiritual senses demonstrate this notion of the dual reality: the corporeal and spiritual person immersed in the visible and invisible world.

39 Cf. Jean D'Apamée, *Dialogue* 6,78; Lavenant, *Dialogues*, 116.

40 René Lavenant translates as follows: "Nous sommes appelés à l'espérance! Que notre pensée ne s'arrête pas à ce monde-ci! Nous devons quitter en esprit ce lieu-ci!". Jean D'Apamée, *Dialogue* 6,81; Lavenant, *Dialogues*, 119.

The purpose of biblical citations in the dialogues is argumentative in John of Apamea's methodology,[41] since Scripture provides the Syrian monk a stepping stone from which to reflect upon the supernatural realities that will be completely manifested and discernible in the world to come. Thus John, in his theological discourses, intrinsically relates the emphasis on the soul's senses to the notion of the eschatological times when God will be completely revealed to humanity. He does not, however, deny God's divine manifestations to humanity in the present moment, which implies the ability of every person to perceive, through the soul's senses, the invisible reality of God in the currently existing world. The presence of God has already been made manifest in human history, yet not in its entirety. Hence, he highlights the present reality as an obstacle that must be overcome, emphasizing the corporeal dimension of the person as the obstruction to exercising the spiritual senses, while simultaneously indicating that this physical world also presents itself as an opportunity for purification to every individual who wants to achieve a superior spiritual level.

The second and sixth dialogues with Thomasios summarize the dualistic conception of reality, which also implies an anthropological dichotomy based in the corporeal person who lives either in accord with or in opposition to the spiritual or interior person. This same vision of the world and the human person is also present in the other four dialogues with Thomasios, the two letters also addressed to Thomasios, and the three tractates published by Lavenant. It would therefore be incorrect to generalize the notion of the tripartite anthropological physiognomy to the entirety of the spirituality and writings of John of Apamea, because the tripartite vision of the person is true only for the work attributed to John that has been published by Sven Dedering with the title of *Ein Dialogue über die Seele und die Affekte des Menschen*, previously mentioned in the first and second chapter of this book.[42] Consequently, the dual conception of the world and humanity seems to be the most appropriate and generalized notion utilized to describe the philosophical and theological view of the Syrian monk.[43]

---

41 Cf. 1Cor 13:8b; 15:43; Hebrews 11:40; Ephesians 1:17.18; Deuteronomy 32:39; Psalm 46:11.

42 For the French critical edition of the same work see Irenée Hausherr, ed. et trans., *Jean le Solitaire, Dialogue sur L'âme et les passions des hommes* (Roma: Pontificium Institutum Orientalium Studiorum, 1939).

43 For a critical position regarding these writings see L. van Leijsen, "De driedeling van het geestelijk leven bij Johannes van Apamea," *JECS* 51, no. 3-4 (1999): 220-236. My personal analysis of the anthropological view in the six dialogues with Thomasios, the two letters, and the three tractates published by Strothmann and Lavenant, indicates the notion of a dualistic dimension of the visible and invisible world and the anthropological dichotomy of the corporeal and interior (or spiritual) person.

Chapter IV

Spiritual Exegesis

1. Premise

Following the line of thinking established in the aforementioned dialogues with Thomasios, it is worth noting the following query: Is it possible to apply this notion of the spiritual senses as a key to reading Mark's Gospel? Is it valid to take this kind of approach to the Gospel? The response is affirmative for both questions. It is possible because since the second century with Origen, the notion of the spiritual senses has been related to the practice of *Lectio Divina* of the Sacred Scripture. This kind of biblical reading has therefore been present as part of the Christian tradition for centuries. In that spiritual reading of the Gospels and personal encounter with the kerygmatic narration of Jesus' life, the believer recognizes that the soul already has the capacity to perceive the divine reality of God through his manifestation in the person of Christ.

Spiritual perception manifests itself subtly in the Gospel's narrative through several characters who are able to see beyond the barriers of physicality. This sort of visual perception is typical of Jesus, who sees as God sees. Therefore when, examining Scripture, the believer reads, "Jesus saw the disciples by the shore," what exactly did Jesus "see" in them for him to call them? It must have been more than just the physical sight of some fishermen working. How is it possible that on certain occasions, the author of the Gospel describes Jesus as seeing the faith of a person or group of people? Is he seeing the manifestations of that faith in deeds, or he is truly seeing the inner mystery of the human soul? Additionally, when the demons see Jesus, they immediately make a profession of faith, saying, "You are the son of God." What is the implication of this statement? Are they seeing an ordinary person, a man called Jesus? Or does this mean that they are seeing something more than the simple man who is approaching them? What are they perceiving? By discovering multiple levels of perception immersed in the kerygmatic narrations of the Gospel, the reader, who approaches the sacred text from the standpoint of faith, can find the ground on which to experience in his or her personal life the path of spiritual recognition hidden in the circumstantial and changing world.

The validity of a *Spiritual Exegesis*, using the theological notions of the superior senses of the soul presented in John of Apamea's second and sixth dialogues as a hermeneutical reading key therefore remains a legitimate approach to use when interpreting Mark's text. This method of ancient exegesis offers the reader the opportunity to discover different manifestations of the spiritual senses in a variety of narrative portraits that are presented in the four Gospels. In this particular study, however, the following chapters will focus only on an exegetical reading of Mark's Gospel in order to make evident the portraits of the spiritual sense of *sight* displayed by some characters in the narration, starting with the person of Jesus himself, then the demons, and finishing with the women at the moment of Jesus' crucifixion, burial, and resurrection. Before presenting those results, it is crucial to delineate succinctly the specific grounds of the *Spiritual Exegesis* developed during the Patristic Era.

2. Spiritual Exegesis: From the Literal Meaning to the Theoria

The Scripture, as a deposit of the divine revelation, presents to its reader polyvalent levels of meaning that serve as an everlasting source of spiritual nourishment, for it cannot be exhausted and its message goes beyond the human conventionalities of language and culture. Its comprehension and understanding is universal, reaching every aspect of the human life, and it is an ever present source of personal, psychological, and spiritual growth.

This characteristic of the sacred text was strongly present in the patristic era, for exegetical work then was not limited to the literal aspect and *nuances* of the text. The nature of Scripture pushed the Christian exegetes to arrive at conclusions that covered a broader spectrum, such as theological tractates and reflections that tried to describe the mystery of God and human nature, Christian ethics—or Tropology—as patterns of behavior based upon the person of Jesus, pastoral applications for the life of the community, and instructions regarding the personal development of Christians. The polyvalent semantic levels manifested in the Scripture were presented synthetically in a *stanza* during the thirteenth century by Augustine of Denmark[1] in order to summarize a tradition existing in history of Christianity since the second century. His brilliant verse

1 Also known as Augustine of Dacia who probably died in the year 1282 CE.

states: "Littera gesta docet, quid credas allegoria, moralis quid agas, quo tendas anagogia,"[2] which can be translated as: "The Letter (literal sense) speaks of deeds, Allegory to faith, the Moral how to act, Anagogy our destiny."[3] The literal meaning is the solid ground upon which it is possible to detect the other semantic stages, as well stated by Thomas Aquinas, STh I, 1, 10, ad I:

> The multiplicity of these senses[4] does not produce equivocation or any other kind of multiplicity, seeing that these senses are not multiplied because one word signifies several things, but because the things signified by the words can be themselves types of other things. Thus in Holy Writ no confusion results, for all the senses are founded on one—the literal—from which alone can any argument be drawn, and not from those intended in allegory, as Augustine says in his *Epistle against Vincent the Donatist* from the things said by allegory (Epis. XLVIII). Nevertheless, nothing of Holy Scripture perishes on account of this, since nothing necessary to faith is contained under the spiritual sense which is not elsewhere put forward by the Scripture in its literal sense.[5]

Corresponding to the multiplicity of meanings implied in the revealed content manifested in the written form of the Scripture, it is important to emphasize that in the present study, the literal and spiritual meanings serve as the pivotal semantic levels of interpretation upon which most of the patristic exegetical production is found.

The notion of the semantic levels of the Scripture implies a vertical and spatial dimension in the human psychology. For instance a person might understand the literal semantic level as the "lower" or "basic" meaning that can be found in the text itself that would be easier to grasp because its meaning could be interpreted as "obvious", whereas the spiritual meaning implies a "higher" level of understanding that is connected to the divine mysteries of the person of Christ or

---

2 Innocenzo Gargano, "La Metodologia esegetica dei padri," in *Metodologia dell'Antico Testamento*, ed. Horacio Simian-Yofre (Bologna: Dehoniane, 1995), 205.

3 CCC 118.

4 In this context the term "sense" is intended as semantic level or meaning.

5 Thomas Aquinas, STh I, 1, 10, ad I: "Ad primum ergo dicendum quod multiplicitas horum sensuum non facit aequivocationem, aut aliam speciem multiplicitatis, quia, sicut iam dictum est, sensus isti non multiplicantur propter hoc quod una vox multa significet; sed quia ipsae res significatae per voces, aliarum rerum possunt esse signa. Et ita etiam nulla confusio sequitur in sacra Scriptura, cum omnes sensus fundentur super unum, scilicet litteralem; ex quo solo potest trahi argumentum, non autem ex his quae secundum allegoriam dicuntur, ut dicit Augustinus in epistola contra Vincentium Donatistam. Non tamen ex hoc aliquid deperit sacrae Scripturae, quia nihil sub spirituali sensu continetur fidei necessarium, quod Scriptura per litteralem sensum alicubi manifeste non tradat." Thomas Aquinas, *Summa Theologica* (New York – Boston: Bezinger Brothers, 1947), 7.

the manifestation of the Trinitarian God—the Father, the Son, and the Spirit—through the revealed text.[6] Subsequently, the vertical or hierarchical image of the scriptural *strata* demands extending the meaning beyond a simply literal interpretation according to the intention of the human and divine author of the Scripture.

The spiritual exegesis consists then in an interpretive reading that starts with the letter or literal meaning and moves from there to attain a higher comprehension, arriving at the spiritual semantic level or *theoria* after the systematic study of the text. These two semantic levels, the literal and the spiritual, became two scientific exegetical approaches in antiquity that were easily contrasted as opposites. Such a distinction has the great risk of being too simplistic, since both approaches have an essential common ground, which is the written text, that is to say the written divine word. In antiquity two schools of exegesis essentially embodied these two approaches: the School of Antioch which developed the historical approach of the text based upon the validity of the critical literal meaning, and the School of Alexandria, which focused predominantly on the allegorical reading of the Scripture.[7]

Taking two emblematic representatives as examples of consideration from each theological path, Theodore of Mopsuestia from the School of Antioch, and Origen form the Alexandrian school, we arrive at the conclusion that both methods of interpretation have as a common ground the rhetorical-grammatical study of the text. Their two lines of thought, however, diverge due to the fact that they rely upon two distinct philosophical schools of thought, Platonism and Aristotelianism, both of which were prevalent at that time in the Hellenistic world, along with considerable Stoic influences. The School of Antioch followed the Aristotelian point of view, emphasizing the objective and historical implication of the text in order to discover the intention of the author and the *Sitz im Leben* in which the sacred book was originated; they believed that the manifestations of God to humanity must be understood and analyzed in their respective historical contexts.[8] On the other hand, the Alexandrian school, being influenced by Platonism, read the text according to a dichotomous vision of reality that is grounded in the simultaneous dual existence of physical and spiritual realities.

---

6 Cf. Charles Kannengiesser, ed., *Handbook of Patristic Exegesis* (Leiden – Boston: Brill, 2004), I, 168.206.

7 Cf. Jacques Guillet, "Les exégèses d'Alexandrie et d'Antioche. Conflit ou malentendu?," *RScR* 34 (1947): 257–302; Henri de Lubac, "Typologie et Allegorisme," *RScR* 34 (1947): 180-226.

8 Cf. Thomas Böhm, "Allegory and History," in *Handbook of Patristic Exegesis*, ed. Charles Kannengiesser (Leiden – Boston: Brill, 2004), I, 214-216.218-219.

The methodological exegesis of neither schools can be understood as a systematic presentation of these two philosophical currents. These two philosophical positions provided the intellectual tools needed to construct a more efficient and logical approach to the inspired text. The Antiochian and Alexandrian exegesis use elements and principles established in these philosophical platforms in order to present an original scientific reading of the Scripture. It is worth noting that the Antiochian school acknowledged the fact that there are some passages in Scripture that require a *non-literal* interpretation, and for this reason Theodore of Mopsuestia integrated his historical-literal approach with the notion of "typology." Thus a passage from the Old Testament can be understood as a "typos" or "figure" of the event or person of Christ, since the history of the chosen people of Israel points to its fulfillment in the Christian era.[9] The notion of typology renders the connection between the Old and the New Testament more insightful for exegesis and makes evident the twofold semantic level of the literal sense that *anagogically* leads the believer to the mystery of Christ and the Trinity, that is to say, the spiritual meaning. In this manner the biblical text opens to a spiritual dimension that traverses the boundaries of the testaments in order to serve as a source of divine knowledge for the present Christian situation.[10]

The great opposition between these two approaches can be considered a misunderstanding, that tended to be exaggerated and generalized through a naive understanding of these two schools, since both had built their interpretations upon the solid foundation of the written word. The allegorical approach, typical of the Alexandrian School with Origen as its most eminent representative, was so successful and fruitful in attacking the Gnostic exegesis with the same intellectual tools that it promoted a *sequela* of inflated Allegorism, which in turn provoked the antagonistic reaction of the School of Antioch.

A balanced position between both exegetical currents was not always successful on both sides. However, the Cappadocian fathers, among whom it is worth mentioning Gregory of Nyssa, arrived at a higher level of theological reflection and also achieved a more balanced and integrative approach to Scrip-

---

9 Regarding the notion of Typology in Theodore of Mopsuestia see Manlio Simonetti, *Lettera e/o Allegoria. Un contributo alla storia dell'esegesi patristica* (Roma: Institutum Patristicum Augustinianum, 1985), 156-201. Regarding the exegetical methodology of Theodore of Mopsuestia see Rowan A. Greer, *Theodore of Mopsuestia. Exegete and Theologia* (London: Faith Press, 1961), 112-131; Camillus Hay, "The Christology of Theodore of Mopsuestia," *ABR* 9 (1961): 43–45; Robert C. Hill, "His Master's Voice: Theodore of Mopsuestia on the Psalms," *Heythrop Journal* 45, no. 1 (2004): 40-53; Frederick G. McLeod, "Theodore of Mopsuestia Revisited," *ThS* 61, no. 3 (2000): 447-480; Böhm, "Allegory and History," 228-232.

10 Cf. Böhm, "Allegory and History," 219-220; Simonetti, *Lettera e/o Allegoria*, 168.

ture. According to Gargano's point of view, Gregory of Nyssa was the first among the Cappadocians to be convinced of the strict unity between a sound profession of faith in Christ, God's mysteries, a pastoral experience of faith, and a methodological exegesis of the Scripture.[11] The exegetical studies of Gregory of Nyssa are accompanied by a protreptic and pastoral aspect that seeks to fertilize the soul of every person who wants to grow in the love of Christ. As examples of his writings, "De vita Moysis"[12] and "Homilies on the Canticle of Canticles" can be mentioned.[13] Both dimensions, the spiritual life of faith and a scientific study of Scripture, are in unison, forming a harmonious manifestation of orthodox and mystical theology. As a result of his well-balanced presentation of Scriptural interpretation with a rhetorical exhortation applied to the pastoral education of his time, it is possible to consider this Cappadocian father as one of the most solid theologians of the fourth century who gives us even today an example of a congruent study and interpretation of Scripture.

3. Allegorism and Anagogy

Origen, speaking about the nature of God in *De Deo*, which is in his first book of the *Peri Archon*, clearly establishes the need to interpret, but not literally, the passages that describe God with a physical body or through anthropomorphic images. The anthropomorphism of God was not accepted by Origen, but without denying the value of the written text, he affirmed the need for openness to a higher level of understanding regarding the passages that present God in a limited and circumstantial form. In other words, for Origen, it was unacceptable to acknowledge Yhwh as God in bodily terms. Origen recognized the richness of the literal sense from an etymological point of view. But he also acknowledged the danger of pure literalism in the study of the Scripture since that can lead to dangerous misunderstandings of the salutary message according to the scriptural mode of communication, closing the doors to the spiritual understanding of the passages. Therefore, an absolutely literalistic reading of the Scripture betrays the message of salvation contained in it. In his *Peri Archon*, Origen asserts:

> I know that some will attempt to say that, even according to the declarations of our own Scriptures, God is a body, because in the writings of Moses they find it said,

11 Cf. Gargano, "La Metodologia esegetica," 199.

12 Gregory of Nyssa, *De vita Moysis*, ed., Herbert Musurillo (Leiden: Brill, 1964).

13 Regarding this work of Gregory of Nyssa see Innocenzo Gargano, *La Teoria di Gregorio di Nissa sul Cantico dei Cantici. Indagine su alcune indicazioni di metodo esegetico* (Roma: Pontificium Institutum Studiorum Orientalium, 1981), 95-244; also see Böhm, "Allegory and History," 221-224.

that "our God is a consuming fire," and in the Gospel according to John, that "God is a Spirit, and they who worship Him must worship Him in spirit and in truth." Fire and spirit, according to them, are to be regarded as nothing else than a body. Now, I should like to ask these persons what they have to say respecting that passage where it is declared that God is light; as John writes in his Epistle, "God is light, and in Him there is no darkness at all." Truly He is that light which illuminates the whole understanding of those who are capable of receiving truth, as is said in the thirty-sixth Psalm, "In Thy light we shall see light." For what other light of God can be named, "in which any one sees light," save an influence of God, by which a man, being enlightened, either thoroughly sees the truth of all things, or comes to know God Himself, who is called the truth? Such is the meaning of the expression, "In Thy light we shall see light", i.e., in Thy word and wisdom which is Thy Son, in Himself we shall see Thee the Father. Because He is called light, shall He be supposed to have any resemblance to the light of the sun? Or how should there be the slightest ground for imagining, that from that corporeal light any one could derive the cause of knowledge, and come to the understanding of the truth? If, then, they acquiesce in our assertion, which reason itself has demonstrated, regarding the nature of light, and acknowledge that God cannot be understood to be a body in the sense that light is, similar reasoning will hold true of the expression "a consuming fire". For what will God consume in respect of His being fire? Shall He be thought to consume material substance, as wood, or hay, or stubble? And what in this view can be called worthy of the glory of God, if He be a fire, consuming materials of that kind? ... It is the custom of sacred Scripture, when it wishes to designate anything opposed to this gross and solid body, to call it spirit, as in the expression, "The letter killeth, but the spirit giveth life," where there can be no doubt that by "letter" are meant bodily things, and by "spirit" intellectual things, which we also term "spiritual."[14]

---

14 Origen, *Peri Archon*, I,1–2. The following is the original text in PG 11:121–122: "Scio quoniam conabuntur quidam etiam secundum Scriptures nostras dicere Deum corpus esse, quoniam inveniunt scriptum esse apud Moysem quidem: 'Deus noster ignis consumens est'; in Evangelio vero secundum Joannem: 'Deus spirtus est, et eos qui adorant eum, in spiritu et veritate oportet adorare'. Ignis vero et spiritus non aliud apud eos quam corpus esse putabitur. Quos interrogare volo quid dicant de eo quod scriptum est, quia Deus lux est, sicut Joannes in Epistola sua dicit: 'Deus lux est, et tenebrae non sunt in eo'. Ista nempe lux est, quae illuminat omnem sensum eorum, qui possunt capere veritatem, sicut in XXXV psalmo dicitur: 'In lumine tuo videbimus lumen'. Quid enim aliud lumen Dei dicendum est, in quo quis videt lumen, nisi virtus Dei, per quam quis illuminatus vel veritatem rerum omnium pervidet, vel ipsum Deum cognoscit qui veritas appellatur? tale est ergo quod dicitur: 'In lumine tuo videbimus lumen'; hoc est, in Verbo et sapientia tua, qui est Filius tuus, in ipso te videbimus Patrem. Numquidnam quia lumen nominatur, simile putabitur solis hujus lumini? Et quomodo vel levis aliquis dabitur intellectus, ut ex isto quis corporali lumine causam scientiae capiat, et veritatis inveniat intellectum? (2) Si ergo acquiescunt huic assertioni nostrae quam de natura luminis ipsa demosntrativit ratio, et fatentur non posse corpus intelligi Deum secundum luminis intellectum, similis quoque ratio de igne consumente dabitur. Quid enim consumet Deus

Hence the literal sense must be complemented with a higher level of understanding found in the Spirit inspired-text, where the hermeneutical key must be the person of Christ and the inscrutable mystery of God. Accordingly the dichotomy, influenced by the Platonic conception of the reality[15] and now applied to the world of the Scripture, is clear. In Origen the dual notion of the literal and spiritual semantic levels is crucial for his understanding of the sacred text that is *per se* veiled by its written form. The written language being the privileged manner of the preservation and transmission of the divine content through centuries, also becomes the cloth that covers the mystery contained in the Scripture. Consequently, Origen talks about the need to "unveil" the true meaning of the Scripture, that is to unearth the deeper meaning of the text and make it evident with the intent to mature in the spiritual knowledge of God.

> The apostle, moreover, says, "Even unto this day, when Moses is read, the veil is upon their heart: nevertheless, when it shall turn to the Lord, the veil shall be taken away: and where the Spirit of the Lord is, there is liberty". For so long as any one is not converted to a spiritual understanding, a veil is placed over his heart, with which veil, i.e., a gross understanding, Scripture itself is said or thought to be covered: and this is the meaning of the statement that a veil was placed over the countenance of Moses when he spoke to the people, i.e., when the law was publicly read aloud. But if we turn to the Lord, where also is the Word of God, and where the Holy Spirit reveals spiritual knowledge, then the veil is taken away, and with unveiled face we shall behold the glory of the Lord in the holy Scriptures.[16]

---

secundum hoc quod ignis est? Nunquidnam putabitur consumere materiam corporalem, ut est lignum, vel fenum, vel stipula? et quid in hoc dignum Dei laudibus dicitur, si Deus ignis est hujusmodi materias consumens? ... consuetudo est Scripturae sanctae cum aliquid contrarium corpori huic crassiori et solidiori designare vult, spiritum nominare, sicut dicit: 'Littera occidit, spiritus autem vivificat'. In quo sine dubio per literam corporalia significat, per spiritum intellectualia, quae et spiritalia dicimus."

15 For the Myth of the Cave in Plato see The Republic book VII: Plato, *The Republic*, ed. et trans. Desmond Lee (New York: Penguin Classics, 2007).

16 Origen, *Peri Archon*, I, 2. Original text in PG 11:122: "Apopstolus quoque dicit: 'Usque in hodierum cum legitur Moyses velamen est positum super cor eorum; cum autem coversus fuerit quis ad Dominum, auferetur velamen; ubi autem Spiritus Domini, ibi libertas'. Donec enim quis non se converterit ad intelligentiam spiritalem, est positum velamen super cor ejus, quo velamine, id est intelligentia crasiore, Scriptura ipsa velari dicitur vel putatur; et hoc est quod ait superpositum esse velkamen vultui Moysi eum loqueretur ad populum, id est cum lex vulgo recitaretur. Si autem convertamus nos ad Dominum, ubi est et Verbum Dei, et ubi Spiritus sanctus revelat scientiam spiritalem, tunc auferetur velamen, et tunc revelata facie in Scripturis sanctis gloriam Domini speculabimur." Also see *Peri Archon* III, 6:1; IV, 1:6; IV, 2:8.

This conception constitutes the essential platform of the Allegorical methodology developed by Origen, which is the representative scriptural approach of the Alexandrian school. The Greek term allegory, ἀλληγορία, has the basic meaning of a description of one thing under the image of another, which is a derivative of the verb ἀλληγορέω which means "to speak so as to imply something other than what is said."[17] The term *Allegory* is in fact a composite term, and it is derived from the expression ἀλλά ἀγορεύω, which can be translated as "I say or declare something else in a public speech." The verb ἀγορεύω literally means to speak in the assembly, or ἀγορά, in order to counsel an audience.[18] The notion of allegory indicates that a text can hide a deeper meaning, one which needs to be declared or proclaimed to the audience of believers who do not have access to its deeper meaning. The key to opening the different doors of meaning in the sacred text is the mystery of the Logos: Jesus Christ. The need for this kind of exegesis has a rich attestation. Apart from the Alexandrian School, there exist exegetical writings that provide extra-biblical evidence to demonstrate that this method had been in practice since the fifth and fourth century BCE.[19]

The allegorical method assumes as a principle that the passage or written story intends to say something more than what is obvious in the literal wording. According to this assumption, the exegete must discover the mystical meaning that was intended by the divine author of the Scripture. The literal semantic level is therefore only the starting point of the scriptural education for the one who wants to grow in the knowledge of God.

In an effort to propose an organic theological and exegetical presentation, Origen , in his *Peri Archon* IV, 2:4, tries to harmonize the mystical significance of Scripture with the threefold division of meanings in the analogy of the tripartite Pauline division of the human person. According to Origen's notion, the division of a person into body, soul, and spirit corresponds to three kinds of Christians: the *simpliciores* (*incipiens*), the *progedientes*, and the *perfecti*. Subsequently, the Alexandrian master also analogically applies the tripartite anthropological classification to the three semantic levels of the Scripture which are, respectively, the literal, moral, and spiritual levels.[20] The analogy can be more clearly seen in the following schema:

---

17 Liddell–Scott, "ἀλληγορέω," 35.

18 Liddell–Scott, "ἀγορεύω," 7; Böhm, "Allegory and History," 248.

19 BAGD, "ἀλληγορέω," 39; Böhm, "Allegory and History," 248–250; Friedrich Büchsel, "ἀλληγορέω," *TDNT* I, 260–262.

20 Cf. Manlio Simonetti, *Biblical Interpretation in the Early Church. An Historical Introduction to Patristic Exegesis*, trans. John A. Hughes (Edinburgh – New York: T&T Clark, 1994), 42–43.

Human Person: Body, Soul, and Spirit.
Christians: Simpliciores (incipiens), Progredientes, and Perfecti.
Scripture: Literal meaning, Moral meaning, and Spiritual meaning.

This hermeneutical criterion was not successful in terms of academic organization for the Alexandrian school, for it created more complications in Origen's own exegetical works in matters of ascertaining a categorization of the semantic levels or stages that can be identified in his exegesis. One of the problems in creating an organized classificatory system resides in the fact that Origen was emphasizing different aspects or levels of meaning according to the nature of the text. In this respect, it is important to remember that for Origen, exegetical approaches to the sacred texts cannot be treated as mathematical formulae that fit every situation identically every time they are applied. The Alexandrian exegete was aware that every pericope has its own life and theological fluidity. However, it is also crucial to keep in mind that his most basic principle of the dichotomy in Scripture is a predominant theme in his writings. His dichotomous conception was not merely a copy of the Platonic vision of reality, manifested in Plato's myth of the cave, but a Christian notion that takes its root in the mystery of the incarnation of the second person of the Trinity, the Logos who became Jesus, man and God at the same time. Hence, the mystery of the incarnation justifies and substantiates the basic dualistic division between the literal and spiritual sense. The same principle can be observed in the writings of John of Apamea. The common characteristic of these two Christian authors resides in a most effective theological usage of a dichotomous conception that takes place over a more systematic and elaborated tripartite anthropological and scriptural classification. This dualistic notion, in both cases, is more feasibly conceived as being due to the mystery of the incarnation of the Logos than merely a copy of Platonic and Neoplatonic ideas. Origen, in his Homily on Leviticus 1:1, explicitly establishes this essential principle that permeates all his works:

> As "in the last days", the Word of God, which was clothed with the flesh of Mary, proceeded into this world. What was seen in him was one thing; what was understood was something else. For the sight of his flesh was open for all to see, but the knowledge of his divinity was given to the few, even the elect. So also when the Word of God was brought to humans through the Prophets and Lawgiver, it was covered with the veil of the flesh, so here with the veil of the letter, so that indeed the letter is seen as flesh but the spiritual sense hiding within is perceived as divinity. Such, therefore, is what we now find as we go through the book of Leviticus ...[21]

---

21 Origen, *Homilies on Leviticus. The Fathers of the Church*, trans. Gary Wayne Barkley (Washington: Catholic University Press, 1990), 29.

Origen continues to compare analogically the twofold dimension of the incarnation of the Logos and the Scripture with two kind of Christians: the "simple" Christian who stops at the fleshly level of the literal meaning of Scripture, and the "perfect" Christian who ascends to the spiritual level of significance by unveiling the divine meaning hidden beneath the surface of the Scripture.[22] Thus the mystery of the incarnation that implies the hypostatic union of the human nature embodies the analogy of the simple and perfect Christians, who understand respectively the literal and spiritual meaning of the Scripture.

The taxonomy in the three yet sometimes only two levels shows that "these schematizations had only a relative value for Origen,"[23] as Simonetti maintains, since the richness of the sacred text cannot be exhausted, giving endless fruitful meaning in the life of the believer who comes to the well for the nurture and refreshment of the spirit. In fact, the relationship between the Text and the Reader cannot be motionless; on the contrary, it is dynamic, creating a lively process of growth in the understanding of God's communication through the biblical spirituality.

In this kind of methodology, Christ is not just the object of study in the Scripture, but he is also the exegete *par excellence*. He is the one who teaches the believer how to read and interpret the OT from his own point of view. Applying the same exegetical plan, Origen keeps in mind the unity of all Scripture that has its center in Christ. In this manner, the reader-believer proportionally increases his or her knowledge and comprehension of the spiritual mysteries of the Scripture while at the same time deepening his or her intellectual and spiritual relationship with the person of Christ himself.[24]

The allegorical method, as previously highlighted, has the goal of "elevating" a Christian to the spiritual comprehension of the revelation of God in Scripture. The Greek term ἀναγωγή has the basic meaning of "leading up" which is a derivative from the verb ἀνάγω, meaning "to go up" or "to bring up." The word indicates an upward movement in the comprehension of the sacred text when the spiritual meaning is discovered. Accordingly, with the general notion of *anagogy*, this concept or semantic level can be implied in the allegorical methodology as a part of it and as its intention. Hence this "uplifting" of the person can be considered the *anagogy*. The incorporation of such a notion into exegesis can be found in prominent Christian writers such as Origen, Epiphanius, Metho-

22 Cf. Simonetti, *Biblical Interpretation*, 43.

23 Simonetti, *Biblical Interpretation*, 43.

24 Cf. Gargano, "La Metodologia esegetica," 204-205.

dius, and Gregory of Nyssa among other authors in antiquity.[25] The *anagogy* represents the stage where it is possible to experience the contemplation of the celestial things present in the spiritual realm and the divine mysteries to come; this means that the notion implies an eschatological connotation as eloquently expressed in the declaration of John Cassian: "Anagogy leads from spiritual mysteries to more sublime and more sacred secrets of heavens."[26]

The Alexandrian methodology of exegesis was more than only a biblical approach; it truly exhibited a cultural tradition. The intellectual center of Alexandria developed an authentic spirituality, way of living, and understanding of Christianity. The Alexandrian tradition experienced a diverse range of opinion throughout its history, including times of prominence and times of disrepute, but it nevertheless retained its influence in the sphere of Biblical exegesis without losing its significant alliance (or points of contact) with the Greek culture. The vitality of the Alexandrian School subsisted upon the legacy of Origen himself. For this reason, during the fourth and fifth century, it suffered due to the impact of the Origenist controversies and the progressive emergence of the Monophysite debate.[27] By this point the Alexandrian school had sacrificed much of its traditional Origenist inheritance. Another contributing factor to the decadence of the Alexandrian School was the reaction of the Antiochene Literalism, which became a constant attack to the school of Alexandria, provoking an exaggerated Allegorism that emerged under the inspiration of Origen's tradition.

During the tumultuous fourth and fifth century, this Christian cultural tradition was still alive when John of Apamea arrived in Egypt, where he received his Hellenistic and Christian education from the Alexandrian milieu.[28] In that environment, he immersed himself in the principles of Alexandrian spirituality and its distinct biblical approach. Therefore, in accordance with this *Sitz im Leben*, the Hellenistic Platonic notions helped him to express, in his theological and spiritual dialogues with Thomasios, the twofold reality where the "corporeal person" interacts with the surrounding and immediate world through the bodily senses. Likewise the "interior person"—who can be also called "spiritual"—interacts with the spiritual reality hidden in the immediate world through his or her spiritual senses, to the point of arriving at knowledge of the divine mysteries

25 For a more complete list of the works of the Christian authors mentioned above regarding the assimilation of the notions of allegory and anagogy see Böhm, "Allegory and History," 257.

26 "Anagogia vero de spiritalibus mysteriis ad sublimiora quaedam et sacratiora caelorum secreta cvonscendens." John Cassian, *Collatio* 14,c. VIII (SC 54:190) in Böhm, "Allegory and History," 257.

27 Cf. Simonetti, *Biblical Interpretation*, 110-111.

28 Cf. Lavenant, *Dialogues*, 21.

of God and having a glimpse of the enigma of the world to come. The influence of the Alexandrian Christian Tradition permeates the spiritual conversations of John of Apamea, being a significant cultural background for the understanding of his theology and reading of Scripture. This also justifies the approach of the spiritual exegesis from the same background of the Syrian monk, providing to us a hermeneutical reading key to detect the spiritual seeing in Mark's narrative according to John's theological and scriptural reflections.

4. Patristic Exegesis of Mark's Gospel

During the patristic period, Mark's Gospel received little attention as an individual literary work. Part of the reason for this underestimated approach resides in the literary richness expressed in the great details, vivacity, and theological meanings of the other Synoptic Gospels and John's writings, which were more than sufficient for the patristic meditations and elucidations. However, anyone with the mindset of a scholar can find among several patristic writers particular attention given to various aspects of Mark's Gospel.

The first one to address the importance of Mark's Gospel was Papias, Bishop of Hierapolis in Phrygia during the years 60–130 CE. Papias' concern was the authorship and authority of the Gospel. He affirms that Mark was the interpreter of Peter, thereby indicating that the Markan Gospel preserves one of the earliest attestations of Peter's preaching, manifesting a Petrine authority in its narrative, and an ancient experience of the faith in Christ. The affirmations of the Bishop of Hierapolis are preserved by Eusebius of Caesarea in his *Historia Ecclesiastica* 3.39.14–15:

> But now we must add to the words of his (Papias) which we have already quoted the tradition he gives in regard to Mark, the author of the Gospel. It is in the following words: "This also John the Presbyter said: Mark, having become the interpreter of Peter, wrote down accurately, though not indeed in order, whatever he remembered of the things said or done by Christ. For he neither heard the Lord nor accompanied him, but afterward, as I said, he was in company with Peter, who used to offer teaching as necessity demanded, but with no intention of giving a connected account of the Lord's discourses. So Mark committed no error in thus writing some single points as he remembered them. For upon one thing he fixed his attention: to leave out nothing of what he had heard and to make no false statements in them."[29]

29 Eusebius, *Historia Ecclesiastica* 3.39.14-15 (NPNF 2,1:172-173) in *Mark, ACCS NT II*, eds. Thomas C. Oden and Christopher A. Hall (Downers Grove: InterVarsity Press, 2005), xxi–xxii.

The Phrygian tradition[30] upholds as true the following five statements regarding the apostolic authority of Mark's Gospel:

a) Mark interpreted Peter truthfully.

b) Mark's source was Peter himself.

c) The Gospel was not written "in order."

d) Mark himself did not know the Lord.

e) Mark did not leave out anything of importance in his account. He did not lie in his writing.

Clement of Alexandria (*ca.* 150–215 CE) stated that Mark's Gospel displays the written form of the "good news" for the Roman community, confirming the information of the Phrygian tradition. Tertullian, in the same manner, confirms the Roman tradition and the Petrine authority of the Gospel in his work entitled *Against Marcion* 4.2.5. Origen also corroborates the assumption that Mark preserved the preaching of Peter, specifying that the apostle himself instructed and ordered Mark to write it down. Following this line of tradition, Origen found 1 Peter 5:13 as a biblical ground for this belief, for there "my son" is written in reference to Mark.[31] Irenaeus, in his *Adversus Haereses* 3.1.1, states the same tradition, but he adds that Mark wrote the Gospel right after Peter's death.[32] Augustine, however, in his *De Consensu Evangelistarum* 1.2, establishes Matthew's priority, meaning that he held that the Matthean account was the first Gospel to be written and that Mark followed after him, containing most of the information already found in Matthew's version.[33]

Jerome, contra Irenaeus, affirms the following: "Peter had inspected and approved Mark's report, and that Mark took Peter's Gospel to Alexandria and died there as first bishop of Alexandria."[34] Consequently Jerome, highlighting the importance of this Gospel, ascribes its authority to Peter himself in his *Lives of Illustrious Men* 1: "Then too the Gospel according to Mark, who was his (Peter's) disciple and interpreter, is ascribed to him (Peter)."[35] Regarding the com-

30 Cf. Oden and Hall, *Mark*, xxii.

31 Cf. Oden and Hall, *Mark*, xxiii.

32 Cf. David L. Balás and Jeffrey Binham, "Mark," in *Handbook of Patristic Exegesis. The Bible in Ancient Christianity*, ed. Charles Kannengiesser (Leiden – Boston: Brill, 2004), I, 343.

33 Cf. Oden and Hall, *Mark*, xxvii.

34 Oden and Hall, *Mark*, xxvi.

35 Cf. *NPNF* 2, 3:36, in Oden and Hall, *Mark*, xxvi, note 16.

ments and sermons based upon the stories of Mark's Gospel, Jerome presented the fullest and most extant treatments of this Gospel among the fathers of the Church. But there are also fragments of comments on Mark's Gospel attributed to Theodore of Mopsuestia, and several sermons on selected passages of Mark can also be ascribed to Augustine, John Chrysostom, Peter Chrysologus, and Gregory the Great.[36]

The following list functions as an illustrative and didactic aid in order for the reader of this book to have a panoramic view of the patristic works on Mark's Gospel for future growth in the area of the patristic understanding of this kerygmatic account. The bibliographical elenchus, indicating the most undisputed patristic works on the Markan Gospel, has been proposed by David L. Balás and Jeffrey Binham. It is worth noting the brevity of Mark's list when compared with the copious patristic works regarding the Gospels of Matthew, Luke, and John.[37]

Jerome (Pseudo-Chrysostom), *Tractatus 10 in Marci Evangelium* and *Homilies on the Gospel of Mark*;[38] Pseudo-Jerome, *Expositio Evangelii secundum Markum*, *The First Commentary on Mark*, and *Commentarius in evangelium secundum Marcum*;[39] Augustine, *Sermons* (from the Gospel of Mark) and *Sermons 94A–147A* on the NT;[40] John Chrysostom, *Sermons* (from the Gospel of Mark);[41] Peter Chrysologus, *Sermons* (from the Gospel of Mark);[42] Theodore of

36 Cf. Balás and Binham, "Mark," 343.

37 See Balás and Binham, "Mark," 348-353. Regarding the list on Mark's Gospels see Ibid., 350-351.

38 Cf. Jerome (Pseudo-Chrysostom), *Tractatus 10 in Marci Evangelium*, ed. D. G. Morin (Turnhout: Brepols, 1958); CCSL 78:449-500; Id., "Homilies on the Gospel of Mark," in *The Homilies of St. Jerome*, trans. M. L. Ewald (Washington: CUA Press 1964); FC 57:121-192.

39 Cf. Pseudo-Jerome, *Expositio Evangelii secundum Markum*, ed. Michael Cahill (Turnhout: Brepols, 1997), CCSL 82; Id., *The First Commentary on Mark: An Annotated Translation*, trans. Michael Cahill (New York: Oxford University Press, 1998); Id., "Commentarius in evangelium secundum Marcum," in *PL* 30:589-644.

40 Cf. Augustine, "Sermons" (from the Gospel of Mark), in *PLS* 2:424-427; *PL* 38:581-591; 1104-1107; 1112-1115; 1126-1133; Id., "Sermons" (from the Gospel of Mark), in NPNF 1, 6:406-413, trans. R. G. MacMullen and ed. Philip Schaff; Id., "Sermons 94A–147A on the NT", in *The Works of Saint Augustine: A Translation for the 21st Century*, trans. Edmund Hill (Brooklyn, NY: New City Press, 1992), 24-39.

41 Cf. PG 51:31-40; PG 58:603-610; 757-767.

42 Cf. Peter Chrysologus, "Sermons" (from the Gospel of Mark), ed. Alexandre Olivar (Turnhout: Brepols, 1975); CCSL 24:102-105; 122-127; 167-172; 182-190; 206-210; 269-273; 284-291; Id., "Sermons" (from the Gospel of Mark), ed. Alexandre Olivar (Turnhout: Brepols, 1981); CCSL 24A: 505-509; 511-516; 617-619; Id., "Sermons" (from the Gospel of Mark), ed. Alexandre Olivar (Turnhout: Brepols, 1982); CCSL

Mopsuestia, *Fragmenta in Marcum*;[43] Pseudo-Theophilus, *Allegoriae in Evangelium secundum Marcum*.[44]

For a variety of patristic texts taken from different patristic commentaries, tractates, sermons or homilies ascribed to the particular verses of Mark's Gospel, the reader can refer to the edition by Thomas C. Oden and Christopher A. Hall in the Ancient Christian Commentary Series, *Mark, ACCS NT II* (Downers Grove: InterVarsity Press, 2005).[45] This work presents the characteristics of a modern *catena aurea*. That means that for each verse of the Markan Gospel, there is a selection of patristic texts related to the meaning of the pericope, indicating an enormous effort by the editors regarding the selection and organization of the Patristic texts included. It has become a valid and solid instrument of reference in the patristic studies of Mark.

24B: 1040-1049; 1054-1058; 1060-1064; 1068-1072; Id., "Sermons" (from the Gospel of Mark), trans., G. E. Ganss (Washington: CUA Press 1953), 3-287; FC 17:75-80; 133-137; 276-282.

43 Cf. PG 66:713-716.

44 Cf. PLS 3:1308-1312.

45 Also for another list of patristic sermons and homilies on Mark's Gospel, see: Hermann Josef Sieben, *Kirchenväterhomilien zum Neuen Testament: ein Repertorium der Textausgaben und Übersetzungen, mit einem Anhang der Kirchenväterkommentare* (Steenbrugis: Abbatia S. Petri, 1991), 69-71.

Part Two
Mark's Gospel

Chapter V

Mark's Vocabulary: The Literal Semantic Level

In English the most common verb for visual perception is *to see*, but that is not the only one. There is a spectrum of terms employed to express different nuances and levels of seeing according to specific circumstances that are used in daily colloquial communication, such as to observe, to watch, to look at, to examine, to catch sight of, etc. The same phenomenon can serve as an analogy to the Greek koiné, where one can find a rich variety of vocabulary employed to identify different semantic levels of visual perception. Among these, three verbs are quite prevalent in Mark's Gospel: Horáō, Blépō, and Theōréō.

The methodology applied to the sacred texts of Mark entails the usage of a synchronic approach of narrative and semantic analysis.[1] This approach possesses as a hermeneutical ground the notion of the spiritual senses, especially *spiritual seeing*, as the key to reading Scripture according to the dialogues of John of Apamea.

The reader can examine the Canonical Greek text[2] in its final form using the different verbs for visual perception as the linguistic criteria, taking into account the context, subject, and object of perception for the verb of seeing. This analysis will emphasize the common semantic level of the verbs of visual perception intended by the author in keeping with the internal evidence in Mark's narrative. For this purpose, it is necessary to start by determining the basic or standard definitions of the verbs used by the author to indicate visual perception and then to study three specific portraits of seeing that show an unambiguous metaphysical or spiritual notion of seeing, as it is in the case of Jesus, the demons, and the women.

---

1 Cf. James L. Resseguie, *Narrative Criticism of the New Testament. An Introduction* (Grand Rapids, MI: Baker Academic, 2005), 17-21.

2 The text used is the Nestle – Aland, *Novum Testamentum Graece* (28th edition; Berlin: Deutsche Bibelgesellschaft, 2012).

1. Horáō (ὁράω)

Horáō is a transitive verb that implies the physical sense of perception which is "to see, to perceive, to catch sight of" (Matt 24:30), "to go to see or visit" (Heb 13:23), or to experience and to witness something. It is the basic action of seeing with the bodily eyes but additionally entails the act of seeing with the mind, that is, to perceive or to know.[3] As an intransitive verb, it has the nuance of looking at someone (John 19:37), but one could predominantly apply it in warnings and instructions to meanings such as "to look out for, watch out, be on guard against," e. g. Matt 16:6; 18:10; 27:4.[4]

Horáō is the most common verb for seeing employed in the New Testament. It appears a total of 350 times in the Gospels, Acts, and Revelation. In Mark, *horáō* appears a total of 59 times including its derivatives.[5]

The second aorist of *horáō*, *eiden*, is worth mentioning, for it bears the following meanings: a perception by sight (Matt 2:2), to become aware of, to feel (Matt 27:54), as well as to take note by observation, to consider, to pay attention to, to look at (Rom 11:22). Mark uses *eiden* five times to describe exclusively Jesus' act of seeing: Mark 1:10.16.19; 2:14; 6:34.

2. Blépō (βλέπω)

Blépō, like *horáō*, also has as its basic meaning to see or to look at. It denotes the sense of being able to see as distinct from blindness (Matt 12:22; 15:31; Mark 8:23; Luke 7:21). *Blépō*, connoting the idea of someone who sees and discerns with the bodily eye, also includes the following nuances: to be possessed of sight, to have the power to see, to turn the eyes towards anything (to look at, to look upon, to gaze at), to perceive by the senses, to feel, to discover by use, to know by experience. Additionally, the meaning of comprehension and intellectual perception of ethical behavior is implied in this verb.[6]

Metaphorically, the verb *blépō* signifies the following: to see with the mind's eye, to have the power of understanding, to discern mentally, to observe, to perceive, and to discover something or somebody to the point that it can evoke an emotional response, to feel, to turn the thoughts or direct the mind to a

3 Cf. BAGD, 577-577.

4 Cf. Wilhem Michaelis, "ὁράω," *TDNT* V, 340-342.

5 According to my statistics of the verb horáō in the literary corpus of the Gospels in the Greek text of Nestle–Aland (28th ed.) the verb has the following presences: Matthew: 72 times, Mark: 59 times, Luke: 85 times, and John: 70 times.

6 Cf. Moulton and Milligan, "βλέπω," 113; Liddell–Scott, "βλέπω," 131.

thing or person, to consider, to look at, to weigh carefully, to examine, to look deeply into, to see through or to become aware of the essence.[7] In relation to the mental functions, the verb implies directing one's attention in order to take notice of something or somebody, to regard or consider (1 Cor 1:26), to discover, to find, to become aware of (Rom 7:23). In addition to these notions, it can also mean to take warning, e.g.: "watch, beware, be on guard or take heed" as it appears in Mark 13:9 (*blépete*).

Mark prefers to make use of *horáō* rather than *blépō* in order to speak more explicitly of Jesus' seeing; nevertheless, *blépō* and its compound forms occur a total of 32 times in Mark's Gospel, of which 9 appearances refer to the action of seeing by Jesus, i.e.: Mark 3:5.34; 5:32; 6:41; 7:34; 10:21.23.27; 11:11.[8]

3. Theōréō (θεωρέω)

Theōréō has the connotation of mentally or spiritually viewing something or somebody in order to consider it. This notion indicates a physical perception that does not stop in the superficiality of the circumstantial events or persons but rather penetrates through it to a deeper level of insight. Therefore *theōréō*, besides having the basic meaning of seeing by being a spectator and looking, observing, and perceiving with the physical eyes, also has the *nuance* of perception by the mind or spirit, signifying one who can perceive the true nature of the gods as already established in Greco-Roman milieu. Sallustius gives us an illustrative example of the spiritual implication of the verb when he applies it to signify the perception of the true nature of the gods in his work περί θεῶν και Κόσμου. He states: τὰς οὐσίας τῶν θεῶν θεωρεῖτε[9] indicating the following idea: "perceive (or contemplate) the substance of the gods" which can be seen with the intellect (nous) since the physical perception never would be able to observe the divine nature. The sublime connotation of the spiritual perception embodied in *theōréō* turns out to be a special gift of the one sent by God. It is a seeing possible only to one who believes, e.g., John 14:17.19; 17:24.[10]

---

7 Cf. BAGD, 143-144.

8 The verb Blépō has the following presences in the Greek text of Nestle–Aland (28th ed.): Matthew: 26 times, Mark: 32 times, Luke: 27 times, and John: 24 times.

9 Sallustius, περί θεῶν και Κόσμου, chapter 4, paragraph 4,24. ed. A. D. Nock (Cambridge,UK: Cambridge University Press, 1926).

10 Cf. BAGD, 360.

Theōréō has a modest presence in Mark's Gospel, appearing only seven times.[11] The subjects of this verb in the Markan narrative are worth mentioning: Jesus' seeing is described twice with this verb in Mark 5:38; 12:41; the Demons once in Mark 3:11; the crowd seeing the demoniac who had been cured in Mark 5:15, and the women three times in Mark 15:40.47; 16:4.

4. Dictionary versus the Context

It is widely acknowledged in scholarship that the search of a word in a specialized dictionary is not sufficient in the process of discovering the true meaning of the term in the sentence according to the intention of the author who needed to discern which words to use for a specific passage. A simple example from modern life can illustrate this point of view regarding the biblical text. A young person who wants to learn English comes to the United States, and while he/she is walking on the street, hears some other young people saying "What a cool car!". Immediately he/she picks his/her dictionary up and searches for the word "cool," finding the following definition: "moderately cold; neither warm nor cold, fresh, e.g. a rather cool evening, etc." When a native English speaker understands truly the nuance of the colloquialism, he/she realizes that the dictionary's definition does not equate with the intention and meaning of the teenagers, but for the young person who does not speak English, the meaning given by the dictionary is initially problematic. Hence the key element to understanding the true meaning of that term or expression is the context or actual circumstances in which it was spoken. For this reason, the study of the biblical context in which every term appears, helps the reader to determine the nuances and the proper significance the message was intended to have, and in this way the reader uncovers the true meaning that the author had in mind when he was writing the text to a particular community of faith.

With this notion in mind, the reader must not interpret Mark's Gospel as a systematic tractate of the verbs of visual perception where a clear distinction of them is easy to grasp in accordance with the lexicon. Precisely because of the multifaceted aspect of the language in the Gospel, a natural desire for discovery stimulates the exegesis that must be done by the reader in order to detect other semantic levels of the Markan narrative that often escape in a superficial reading of the text.

Of course, this exegetical approach implies a diachronic study of the text, which becomes the real challenge in any biblical study. In our modern times, we

11 The verb theōréō has the following presences in the Greek text of Nestle–Aland (28th ed.): Matthew: 2 times, Mark: 7 times, Luke: 7 times, and John: 24 times.

encounter the difficulty of finding the true meaning of expressions, which, according to their usage, do not correspond to the meanings listed in the official dictionaries, as previously exemplified. Recalling the example given, how much more so is this case when we need to perform the same operation with a language that has not been spoken for over twenty centuries. The cultural and the linguistic gaps are enormous. That is why the main purpose of every exegesis is to discover the semantic levels implied in the texts and to discern which most accurately matches the real intention of the author of the text.

5. A Psychological Approach: *Seeing* and *Seeing as*

The definition of the verb "to see" essentially implies the physical perception of the circumstantial reality that encircles every person. The point is that the physical perception generates emotions, experiences, and knowledge that affect the person in a most profound manner. When a person "sees" a terrific or fantastic event, his or her life can change forever, meaning that the visual perception is connected to the psychology of the person, modifying his or her way of thinking about and considering the surrounding world.

Ludwig Wittgenstein, in his *Philosophical Investigations*, already distinguishes two different usages of the verb "to see."[12] When this verb is used, one implication of this action is the "seeing" of somebody or something, which entails that the object of vision is able to be verified and demonstrated by the physical experience of it, or confirmed by the objective observation of other persons, as for example the observation of the Empire State Building in New York City by thousands of people. It is an object that is verifiable, since many people are "seeing" it.

The other distinction of Wittgenstein is called "seeing as," which is an observation that, unlike the previous one, cannot be verified, since each person will perceive something that can be observed differently by another person, so that the field of physical perception reaches the *subjectivity* of the person who sees an object or other person as a being that calls forth an objectively indemonstrable diversity of emotions, sensations, and experiences. An example is the forms of the clouds in the sky, which may be perceived as a bird or an elephant, depending on what a particular person sees in that specific entity. Another illustration is the changing lights of the Empire State Building during the nights in New York that provoke various effects in each individual according to their personal experiences and cultural background, or might even provoke frustration for

12 Cf. Ludwig Wittgenstein, *Philosophical Investigations*, trans. Gertrude Elizabeth M. Anscombe (New York: Macmillan, 1953), 193.

somebody who is color blind and sees that his friends are amazed by the beauty of the event. The experience of the "seeing as" can be better understood in the field of art appreciation, since one piece of art, a painting of Rembrandt, for example, can motivate and stimulate different aspects of appreciation and perception in each person, causing them to express their interests in the colors or in one color in particular, in the shades, postures of the figures, dimensions, etc.[13] The painting may evoke a different emotional reaction in each person, allowing hidden feelings to surface.

After briefly describing this distinction, it would be a great temptation for the reader to conclude that the "seeing" is objective and real, whereas the "seeing as" is subjective and therefore not real or true. This simplistic conclusion must be considered erroneous, because "when I see a cloud as a camel the experience is as vivid as when I see the cloud itself."[14] Thus the "seeing as" is as real as the objective seeing, with the difference consisting in how to verify each reality in a scientific manner. For the person who experiences particular events or comes into contact with special persons and objects, his or her seeing is so real that it has the potential to transform the life of the one seen radically if what is seen is something extremely influential and important.

The studies of Aesthetics done by Monroe Beardsley complement the previously expounded notion. Beardsley, in order to explain that "X is good because ...", establishes three general canons or criteria of perception. The first is the criterion of *unity* and organization of an object, for example a piece of art. The second is the *complexity* that can be perceived as rich, poor, disturbing, enlightening, mediocre, etc. The third criterion is based upon the notion of intensity which causes a person to experience a situation or object as vivid, forceful, beautiful, graceful, tender, tragic or evil.[15]

Now it is absolutely essential to apply the notions described previously to our field of study. The notion of seeing in Mark's Gospel exhibits the physical action of visual perception, namely, "seeing," but it simultaneously also highlights the subjects of the verbs: Jesus, demons, and the women who see the situations or persons as something that is experienced intensively, matching the third criteria of Beardsley. So when Jesus sees his prospective disciples, he is seeing

13 To have a more complete view regarding these categories, see Ingrid Stadler, "On Seeing As," *Philosophical Review* 67 (1958): 91-94; Walter H. Clark, "Seeing as and Knowing that in Aesthetic Education," in *Aesthetic Concepts and Education*, ed. Ralph A. Smith (Urbana – Chicago – London: University of Illinois Press, 1970), 183-184.

14 Clark, "Seeing as," 184.

15 Cf. Monroe Beardsley, *Aesthetics: Problems in the Philosophy of Criticism* (New York: Harcourt, Brace, 1958), 456.462. For the general conception described see chapter 10 of Beardsley's work. Also see Clark, "Seeing as," 188-190.

them as more than just simple fishermen; he can recognize in them a potentiality that is only perceived by the divine nature of the Logos in the person of Jesus, experiencing these perceptions in a level of consciousness that belongs to God alone in the hypostatic union manifested *in persona Christi*. Almost anyone else would see them as simple fishermen with a low educational level and an insignificant status in society according to a modern point of view. But the Lord sees them differently, seeing each as someone worthy of his calling, personal attention, and consideration. The reality of the *seeing as* of Jesus cannot be objectively verifiable in that precise moment; however, his visual experience of the apostles is as real as their objective existence. History then objectively proved the worth of whatever Jesus saw in them by their martyrdom.

The demons see Jesus as the Son of the most high God (Ἰησοῦ υἱὲ τοῦ θεοῦ τοῦ ὑψίστου Mark 5:7) or the holy one of God (ὁ ἅγιος τοῦ θεοῦ Mark 1:24), namely, according to his divine nature, which provoked in them an intense reaction that is experienced as forceful, tragic, and awful, since they cannot stand in the presence of God. The women, in the context of the death and burial of Jesus, see the lifeless body of Jesus with the intensity of a tragic event that indelibly marked their lives. It is not just the seeing of a dead body, but the intensity of seeing something experienced in their personal *psyche* as heartbreaking. It is an event that will change the life of anyone who sees it.

With the philosophical and psychological approach to the experience of seeing, the reader can conclude that human experiences lived through a variety of circumstances, go beyond the physical realm to touch the inner psyche of a person. Subsequently, the subjective experience of seeing can be as real and profound as an object that can be perceived by a group of witnesses. The reader must admit then that the psychological field serves as the steeping stone in which the spiritual experiences take place. As the body is useful for the psyche, the psyche serves as a connective bridge with the mysterious realm of the spirit. What is experienced in the psyche is as real as the seeing of an object or person confirmable by others; consequently what is experienced by the spiritual senses is as real as the psychological and physical experiences lived through the bodily organs of perception.

The reading of selected pericopes of Mark's Gospel will be delineated by the semantic, narrative, and psychological approach described in order to assert the validity of the spiritual seeing as a real experience. This point of view also confirms the validity of the theological notion of the spiritual senses of John of Apamea as a hermeneutical key to discover this semantic level in the pattern of behavior of the characters in the narrative.

Chapter VI

From Littera to Theoria: Narrative Portrait of Jesus' Seeing

Jesus is the hero of the kerygmatic narrations of the Gospels. Because his actions permeate every single episode of the sacred texts, it would be impractical to study each text where the author implies visual perception of Jesus in the Gospel of Mark. Therefore, for the sake of clarity and academic organization, I have selected texts that serve as proof and confirmation for interpreting verbs of visual perception as spiritual seeing as a probable semantic notion contained in the original intentionality of the author of Mark.

The attestation of the texts is classified into four semantic lines (*Wortfeld*) of action in which the seeing of Jesus serves as the stepping stone for the manifestation of the action of God. Consequently, the seeing of Jesus becomes the first divine action that perceives reality with the intensity of God's sensibility and responsiveness towards humanity. The *Wortfeld* portrayed in the Markan accounts exhibits the following narrative settings:

a) Baptism of the Lord
b) Contexts of calling: Vocatio universalis et specialis
c) Contexts of healing
d) Contemplation

1. The Baptism of Jesus

The first active verb used by the author of Mark to describe Jesus' action in his narrative is the aorist form of the verb ὁράω, εἶδεν, according to the Greek version of the Nestle–Aland 28th edition. The first active seeing of Jesus is placed in the context of his Baptism when he saw (εἶδεν) the heavens torn open and the Spirit descending upon him like a dove (Mark 1:10).

Mark portrays Jesus explicitly as the grammatical *subject* of the verb εἶδεν. The *object* (in the accusative) of his vision turns out to be twofold as one can reads the sequence of the events seen in the narrative: Jesus saw the heavens torn open (σχιζομένους τοὺς οὐρανοὺς 1:10[a]), and the Spirit descending upon him like a dove (τὸ πνεῦμα ὡς περιστερὰν καταβαῖνον εἰς αὐτόν 1:10[b]). This means that the author emphasizes the first thing Jesus sees as being a non-terrestrial reality. Therefore the beginning of his public ministry starts with the exclusive divine manifestation that reveals the Lord's visual and spiritual focus: to look up to heaven, his Father's place, and see the Holy Spirit coming down to his own reality, namely, the one that implies being human. Thus the first seeing of Jesus is metaphysical[1] in the sense that his visual perception goes beyond or through the physical reality that is seen by the bodily sense of sight. The metaphysical seeing crosses the barrier of corporeal limitations in order to see a spiritual reality that goes unnoticed by the natural corporeal eye but is able to be seen by Jesus. The visual experience of Jesus turns out to be exclusive to him because the text of Mark 1:9-11 indicates that only Jesus was capable of seeing this dual celestial reality.[2]

The synoptic reading of this episode highlights the distinctiveness of Jesus' seeing in Mark. A parallel analysis with Matthew 3:16 indicates that only the Spirit of God like a dove descending on him is related exclusively to the seeing of Jesus, not the opening of heavens: "Jesus, when he was baptized, went up directly from the water: and behold, the heavens were opened to him, and he saw (εἶδεν) the Spirit of God descending as a dove, and coming on him." Matthew specifies that it is the Spirit of God (τὸ πνεῦμα τοῦ θεοῦ), while Mark mentions only the Spirit (τὸ πνεῦμα). The heavenly voice accompanying the celestial vision in Mark addresses Jesus exclusively (Σὺ εἶ ὁ υἱός μου ὁ ἀγαπητός, ἐν σοὶ εὐδόκησα Mark 1:11), unlike in Matthew where the voice speaks of Jesus (the Son) in a third person, indicating an implicit audience (Οὗτός ἐστιν ὁ υἱός μου ὁ ἀγαπητός, ἐν ᾧ εὐδόκησα Matt 3:17).

---

1 The expression "metaphysical seeing" derives from the literal etymological combination of two Greek terms: *metá*, a preposition that has, among many other renditions, the significance of "beyond, upon, after, behind", frequent connotation in the Homeric style, and the substantive *physis* which signifies "nature, natural endowment or condition", implying the naturally regulated order of things of the world that can be seen, physical reality that is commonly perceived by the natural senses of perception. Cf. BAGD, 508. 869-870.

2 The context of Mark 1:9-11 does not indicate that others present at the event could perceive the celestial phenomenon.

The difference in the seeing of Jesus as portrayed by the authors of the Synoptic Gospels can also be noticed in Luke 3:21-22, where the author does not make any reference to Jesus' seeing of any of the objects mentioned in Mark: "Now when all the people were baptized, Jesus also had been baptized, and was praying. The sky was opened, and the Holy Spirit descended in a bodily form like a dove on him; and a voice came out of the sky, saying 'You are my beloved Son. In you I am well pleased.'"

If we consider the theory of the four sources regarding the Synoptic problem proposed by Burnett Streeter, Luke's author knew the source of Mark, including the verses of this particular episode.[3] The following question then arises: why did he not follow the Markan text regarding the usage of the verb εἶδεν? Why did he change this particular narrative detail of the Markan narrative? The answer resides in the theological intention of the author. The theological and spiritual notions embodied in the verb εἶδεν are not the same for the authors of Mark and Luke. The Synoptic reading highlights a dynamic work of redaction in which each of the evangelists contributes their own theological reflections adapted to the community or audience implied in the kerygmatic narrative.

Extending the comparison to John 1:32-34, the reader realizes that the one who sees the Spirit is John the Baptist; Jesus meanwhile is passive in the scene:

> John testified, saying, "I have seen (Τεθέαμαι) the Spirit descending like a dove out of heaven, and it remained on him. I didn't recognize him, but he who sent me to baptize in water, he said to me, 'On whomever you will see (ἴδῃς) the Spirit descending, and remaining on him, the same is he who baptizes in the Holy Spirit'. I have seen (ἑώρακα) and have testified that this is the Son of God."

The Johannine narrative manifests a different dynamic in visual perception. The one who sees is John the Baptist, who is also the voice that proclaims the utterance in the narrative, and Jesus becomes one of the objects of the visual perception with the Spirit. The identification of the divine nature of Jesus is confirmed by the simultaneous observation of the Holy Spirit descending and remaining on him. Through this observation (seeing) of divine and human entities interrelating concurrently in the event of the baptism, John arrives at the knowledge of the identity of Jesus as the Logos incarnated. The Baptist then is able to transcend from a platform of ignorance—I myself did not know him (οὐκ ᾔδειν αὐτόν 1:33)—to the knowledge of Jesus as the Son of God, the only one who can baptize with the Holy Spirit.

---

3 According to Streeter, Luke shares about 330 verses with Mark. See Burnett Hillman Streeter, *The Four Gospels: A Study of Origins, Treating of the Manuscript of Tradition, Sources, Authorship, and Dates* (London: Macmillan, 1924), 160.

The synoptic and comparative readings offer us significant results that indicate the special treatment of Jesus' seeing according to the unique theological intention of Mark's author.

When analyzing the first object of Jesus' perception in the event of the baptism, the theological background of the notion of "heaven" already portrayed in the Old Testament must be established in order to grasp more accurately the importance of the object described in the Markan narrative as the first thing that Jesus sees. The pericopes of the OT present the notion of "heaven" as the abode of God (Tobit 5:16; Ps 80:14; 123:1; Eccl 5:2; Lam 3:41), as a closed place that only Yhwh can open for an extraordinary intervention or involvement with his people (2 Kgs 7:2.19; Exod 9:23; Ps 78:24; Isa 63:19). It can also entail the conception of a vision that reaches beyond the earthly dimension (Ezek 1:1). Heaven is the permanent residence of Yhwh, from whence he looks down and listens to the cry of his people (Deut 26:15; Ps 80:14; Isa 63:15). The fact, therefore, of seeing the heavens being rent apart (σχιζομένους) encompasses a deep spiritual implication, since this aperture indicates a great intervention of Yhwh that builds a new manner of communication between the divine and the human reality.

The verb used by Mark to qualify the "heavens" is the passive participle σχιζομένους of the verb σχίζω which means to part, to divide, to separate; this term is employed only once more in Mark's Gospel in order to describe the rending (ἐσχίσθη) of the Temple's veil in the context of Jesus' death: καὶ τὸ καταπέτασμα τοῦ ναοῦ ἐσχίσθη εἰς δύο ἀπ' ἄνωθεν ἕως κάτω (Mark 15:38). The selective use of this verb by the author of Mark establishes a symbolic cosmic *inclusio* between the Baptism (1:10) and the death of Jesus.[4] As understood by Juel, the term connotes a radical and new situation: "what is opened may be closed; what is torn apart cannot easily return to its former state."[5] The abyss between Heaven and Earth is surpassed by the Trinitarian love of Father and Son, creating a new way of communication in which the humanity is assumed by the divinity. The heaven torn apart exhibits a new situation that, due to the radical action of love revealed in the incarnation cannot go back to its previous state. In other words, the heavenly door cannot be closed, because the new relationship between the Trinitarian God and humanity cannot exist in the same manner as it existed before the event of Christ. The heavenly door remains open up to the

4 Cf. Stephen Motyer, "The Rending of the Veil; A Markan Pentecost?," *NTS* 33 (1987): 155-157; Howard Jackson, "The Death of Jesus in Mark and the Miracle from the Cross," *NTS* 33 (1987): 22-24; David Ulansey, "The Heavenly veil torn: Mark's Cosmic Inclusio," *Bib* 110, no. 1 (1991): 123-124.

5 Donald Juel, *A Master of Surprise: Mark Interpreted* (Minneapolis: Fortress Press, 1994), 33.

present day, and as a result, this new divine-human interaction completely changes the way humanity relates to God, and vice versa.

The descending of the Spirit (καταβαῖνον, Mark 1:10) creates a vivid contrast with the ascending of Jesus from the water (ἀναβαίνων). When the Greek expression ὡς περιστερὰν is considered the equivalent of an adjective, the narrative qualifies the description of the Spirit as being "as a dove" (ὡς περιστερὰν), symbolically describing a supernatural reality that *per se* is without form and body. Another interpretation of ὡς περιστερὰν is as an adverb, meaning the action of descending as dove-like.[6] This means that the noun in its adverbial connotation describes the Spirit's descending upon Jesus as fluid, delicate, and smooth like a dove flying in the firmament. In the present pericope, we can apply both interpretations, meaning that the Spirit, represented with the purity, innocence, and gentleness of a dove, also descends upon Jesus with the gracefulness of a bird hovering in the sky.

The notion of a "dove" can comprise multiple interpretations or semantic connotations. It has been considered the symbol of all kinds of virtues, and more particularly, its gentleness, innocence, and goodness have inspired diverse pious Christian conceptions through history.[7] In the Christian tradition we find multiple examples of the dove being interpreted as a symbol for the Holy Spirit, with most of them converging in the contemplation of the virtues and divine gift associated by analogy with the qualities of the bird. The reflection of John Chrysostom (349–407 CE) gives us a summary of this tradition of interpretation, according to his prayerful and exegetical approach to the text:

> But why in the form of a dove? The dove is a gentle and pure creature. Since then the Spirit, too, is a Spirit of Gentleness, He appears in the form of a dove, reminding us of Noah, to whom, when once a common disaster had overtaken the whole world and humanity was in danger of perishing, the dove appeared as a sign of deliverance from the tempest, and bearing an olive branch, published the good tidings of a serene presence over the whole world. All these things were given as a type of things to come… In this case the dove also appeared, not bearing an olive branch but pointing to our Deliverer from all evils, bringing hope filled with grace. For this dove does not simply lead one family out of an ark, but the whole world toward heaven at her appearing. And instead of a branch of peace from an olive tree, she conveys the possibility of adoption for all the world's offspring in common.[8]

---

6 Cf. Richard Thomas France, *The Gospel of Mark. A commentary on the Greek Text*, NIGTC (Grand Rapids, MI – Cambridge, UK: Eerdmans, 2002), 78.

7 Cf. William Hendriksen, *The Gospel of Mark*, NTC (Grand Rapids, MI: Baker Book House, 1975), 43-44.

8 John Chrysostom, "Homily 12.3 of the Gospel of St. Matthew," in *NPNF* 1 10:77; *TLG* 2062.152,57.205.25-35, 41-47; also see *GMI* 15, in *Mark. ACCS NT II*, eds. Oden and Hall, 13.

According to the Jewish tradition, the rabbinic interpretation of rûaḥ (רוּחַ) gives the reader an idea that is closer to the biblical mindset manifested in Mark. Rashi, commenting on Gen 1:2, affirms the following: "The Spirit of God was moving: the Throne of Glory was standing in the air and moving on the face of the waters by the Spirit of the mouth of the Holy One, blessed be he, and by his Word like a dove that broods on the nest."[9] In the Midrash Rabbah, Rabbi Simeon ben Zoma expresses the following idea regarding the same text of Genesis: "For it is not written here, and the Spirit of God blew, but hovered, like a bird flying and flapping with its wings."[10] There is strong connection between the rabbinic interpretation of the rûaḥ (רוּחַ) being like a dove (bird) and the portrayal of the dove in Mark's Gospel, since the Spirit of God portrayed as a bird or a dove hovering over the waters is framed in a context of creation. These elements illuminate the specific theological reflections of Mark that lead us to conceive of the Baptism as a new creation in Christ where the Trinitarian presence is seen explicitly and exclusively by Jesus. The celestial voice in Mark 1:11 re-affirms the relationship of love between Father and Son in this new state that assumes the human condition: "and a voice came from heaven: 'You are my beloved Son, in whom I am well pleased' (σὺ εἶ ὁ υἱός μου ὁ ἀγαπητός, ἐν σοὶ εὐδόκησα)."

2. Contexts of Calling: Vocatio Universalis et Specialis

The passages telling the story of the calling of the first disciples demonstrate the special connotation of Jesus' seeing used by the author of the Gospel of Mark that manifests how God sees. In the context of vocation, Jesus' seeing turns out to be the first step in his method of choosing the prospective disciples. Mark indicates Jesus' perception with the aorist εἶδεν, "he saw," in three significant passages:

Mark 1:16: Καὶ παράγων παρὰ τὴν θάλασσαν τῆς Γαλιλαίας *εἶδεν* Σίμωνα καὶ Ἀνδρέαν τὸν ἀδελφὸν Σίμωνος ἀμφιβάλλοντας ἐν τῇ θαλάσσῃ· ἦσαν γὰρ ἁλιεῖς.

Mark 1:19: Καὶ προβὰς ὀλίγον *εἶδεν* Ἰάκωβον τὸν τοῦ Ζεβεδαίου καὶ Ἰωάννην τὸν ἀδελφὸν αὐτοῦ καὶ αὐτοὺς ἐν τῷ πλοίῳ καταρτίζοντας τὰ δίκτυα.

Mark 2:14: Καὶ παράγων *εἶδεν* Λευὶν τὸν τοῦ Ἀλφαίου καθήμενον ἐπὶ τὸ τελώνιον, καὶ λέγει αὐτῷ· ἀκολούθει μοι. καὶ ἀναστὰς ἠκολούθησεν αὐτῷ.

---

9 Israel Abrahams, *Studies in Pharisaism and the Gospels* (New York: Ktav Publishing House, 1967), 49.

10 Harry Freedman and Maurice Simon, eds., *Midrash Rabbah, Genesis* (London: Soncino Press, 1961), 18.

After analyzing the verbal sequence, the change of scenery, the characters that appear or disappear from the scene, and the intradiegetic dialogues, I can identify in these three episodes six common essential characteristics:

1) Jesus is presented as moving: he is walking close by or along the seashore: 1:16.19; 2:13.14. The Markan portrait of Jesus is dynamic and active.[11]

2) The initiative comes from Jesus, not from the persons who are seen. The first main action is expressed with the aorist indicative εἶδεν: "he saw." This particular verbal aspect indicates a completed and unique action of perception in time that is most commonly translated as occurring in the past.[12]

3) The direct object (accusative) of the verb εἶδεν is the person of the disciple being called. What Jesus sees is the individual identified in the narrative by his personal name. The first four disciples are mentioned in pairs of brothers, and they are being called to be part of a different kind of vital kinship. As soon as they answered God's call, their biological brotherhood is transformed into a brotherhood of love in which Jesus is the bond of this new community of faith.[13] The Greek text is precise in putting the personal name first followed by the brotherly qualification: "Simon and Andrew, the brother of Simon" (εἶδεν Σίμωνα καὶ Ἀνδρέαν τὸν ἀδελφὸν Σίμωνος 1:16), "James the *son* of Zebedee, and John his brother" (εἶδεν Ἰάκωβον τὸν τοῦ Ζεβεδαίου καὶ Ἰωάννην τὸν ἀδελφὸν 1:19). As with James, in the case of Levi, Jesus first sees the person, and then the narrative states qualification of his bloodline: "Levi the son of Alphaeus" (εἶδεν Λευὶν τὸν τοῦ Ἀλφαίου 2:14). Jesus' seeing is personal and individualistic. The text does not say what specific uniqueness he sees in these prospective disciples, but it must be something that evades an exterior physical seeing. The sight of God goes beyond the conventionalities of culture and appearances, which is why Jesus can recognize, by means of his scrutinizing sight, the potential greatness of those he calls.

4) Each of the chosen persons was seen in the context of his daily activities: the fishermen were casting their nets into the sea or mending them; the tax col-

---

11 Cf. Joy Palachuvattil, *"He Saw." The Significance of Jesus' seeing denoted by the verb eiden in the Gospel of Mark* (Roma: Editrice Ponificia Univesitá Gregoriana, 2002), 93.

12 Cf. Manuel Guerra-Gómez, *El idioma del Nuevo Testamento. Gramática, estilística y diccionario estadístico del griego bíblico*. Facultad de Teología del Norte de España (Burgos: Ediciones Aldecoa, [4]1995), 288.

13 Cf. James Donaldson, "Called to Follow: A Twofold Experience of Discipleship in Mark," *BTB* 5 (1975): 67-77; Klemens Stock, *Marco. Commento contestuale al secondo Vangelo* (Roma: Edizioni ADP, 2003), 37-38.

lector was sitting at the tax collector's booth. This additional detail continues to demonstrate the divine initiative that reaches the individual circumstances of the disciples.

5) Jesus' calling of the disciples is direct and simple: "Follow Me and I will make you become fishers of men" (δεῦτε ὀπίσω μου, καὶ ποιήσω ὑμᾶς γενέσθαι ἁλιεῖς ἀνθρώπων 1:17), "He called them" (ἐκάλεσεν αὐτούς 1:20), and He said to Levi "Follow Me!" (ἀκολούθει μοι 2:14). The call comes after the seeing, so it must be a consequence of Jesus' visual perception.

6) The reaction to Jesus' calling is positive: leaving everything they had been doing, they followed him. The action of following Jesus—or going after him—is illustrated with a verb in aorist denoting a completed and unconditional action: followed him (ἠκολούθησαν αὐτῷ, 1:18), went away following him (ἀπῆλθον ὀπίσω αὐτοῦ, 1:20), followed him (ἠκολούθησεν αὐτῷ, 2:14).

The brief narrative analysis of the three aforementioned passages indicates that Jesus' seeing happens as the first step in the process of vocation. Therefore the divine seeing becomes metaphysical, and more specifically spiritual, since Jesus can perceive the totality of the person, breaking through the barriers of superficiality imposed by the circumstances and culture. Consequently Jesus' seeing is not a casual look at somebody, or just a simple glance toward people doing their jobs. Jesus' seeing remains personal, attentive, penetrating, and selective. His *seeing as* provoked the *vocatio* primorum *discipulorum*, because his personal visual encounter was experienced according to the sensitivity and profoundness of God, to whom nothing is hidden.

The account of Mark 10:17-22 presents a context of calling (*vocatio*) with a negative outcome that sharply contrasts with the calling of the first five disciples. The pericope talks about an unidentified man (εἷς 10:17), who is very pious, faithful to the Mosaic Law, and happens to have many possessions (γὰρ ἔχων κτήματα πολλά 10:22). The most remarkable and distinctive feature of this narration is the way in which Jesus looked at the man in Mark 10:21-22. The verb employed is participle aorist active of ἐμβλέπω: ἐμβλέψας, which means to look at something or somebody deeply, to see everything plainly, or to have a clear view of everything. Figuratively, it means to look at somebody with penetrating eyes in a spiritual manner, namely the perception proper to spiritual seeing.[14] The participle indicates a verbal aspect of the action of seeing deeply for an extended period of time. It is not just a simple gaze in a singular moment. Jesus was looking intensely into the man's soul and heart to the point that his par-

14 Cf. BAGD, "ἐμβλέπω," 254.

ticular and personal seeing leads to love: "And looking intensely at him, Jesus loved him (Ἰησοῦς ἐμβλέψας αὐτῷ ἠγάπησεν αὐτὸν)" (10:21). It is precisely because of his incessant and profound seeing that Jesus' love for the other man has presented itself at that moment in the unique gift to the chosen one of being called: δεῦρο ἀκολούθει μοι (10:21). But his call required something else that the Lord knew because of his scrutinizing eyes: the wealthy man needed to put God first.

The Lord with one statement touched the radical failure in the seemingly perfect spiritual life of this man, whose center was not completely in God. The answer to Jesus' invitation is graphic and vivid in the Markan narrative: "But his face fell at that saying, and he went away sorrowful (ἀπῆλθεν λυπούμενος), for he was one who had great possessions (γὰρ ἔχων κτήματα πολλα)" (10:22). The wealthy man did not say anything; his reaction is clearly a negative response to Jesus. The action of moving away from the Lord (ἀπῆλθεν) is accompanied with the deepest feeling of sadness (λυπούμενος), which indicates a lack of peace and freedom. Thus the wordless response of the one who has many possesions (ἔχων κτήματα πολλα) turns out to be the antonym to the answer of the *vocatio primorum discipulorum*. The sharp contrast becomes evident in the following comparative reading:

Mark 1:18 καὶ εὐθὺς ἀφέντες τὰ δίκτυα *ἠκολούθησαν αὐτῷ*.

Mark 1:20 καὶ ἀφέντες τὸν πατέρα αὐτῶν Ζεβεδαῖον ἐν τῷ πλοίῳ μετὰ τῶν μισθωτῶν *ἀπῆλθον ὀπίσω αὐτοῦ*.

Mark 2:14 καὶ ἀναστὰς *ἠκολούθησεν αὐτῷ*.

Mark 10:22 *ἀπῆλθεν* λυπούμενος.

In the first three cases, the speechless response consists in the person who is called leaving—ἀφέντες and ἀναστὰς —what he is doing or his family environment in order to follow the one who is calling him. The one who has many possessions directs his life in a radical opposed way to the path of the sequela Christi. His going away (ἀπῆλθεν), therefore, contrasts with the disciples' following (ἠκολούθησαν αὐτῷ / ἀπῆλθον ὀπίσω αὐτοῦ / ἠκολούθησεν αὐτῷ). Jesus' invitation demands perfection and radical self-giving of the chosen person. Matthew 19:21 makes this invitation unequivocal in terms of perfection, and that invitation can be read as an implicit statement in Mark: "if you wish to be perfect (τέλειος), go, sell..."[15]

The pericope demonstrates that Jesus' seeing becomes the first step, or stepping ground, of a new relationship of friendship and commitments, that makes his love explicit, motivating its manifestation in his call (*vocatio*). The conditional requirement of the calling indicates Jesus' spiritual seeing that is manifested in his unambiguous request for what was lacking in the soul of the one who appears to be perfect: "One thing you lack (ἕν σε ὑστερεῖ). Go, sell whatever you have (ὅσα ἔχεις πώλησον), and give to the poor (δὸς [τοῖς] πτωχοῖς), and you will have treasure in heaven; and come, follow me" (Mark 10:21). Although Jesus admires the sincerity and integrity of someone who carefully follows the Law (Torah), he also can see concurrently what is lacking in the person in order to demand of him the indispensable step that would lead him to be acceptable in front of God's eyes. This capacity of perception goes beyond the human faculty of observation. It is the seeing of God, to whom nothing is able to escape being seen, not even the farthest reaches of the human soul.

3. Contexts of Healing

The pericope of Mark 2:1-5 displays a curative context regarding an anonymous man who cannot walk. His paralysis impedes him from approaching the Lord, since his illness isolated him from any kind of normal social life that would allow him to discover the whereabouts of Jesus in town. However, the most important characters in this narration are four anonymous men who, knowing the Lord's proximity, found the house where he was. Then, conscious of the incapacity of the crippled man to come close to Jesus, they exerted the effort required to carry him.

Despite the obstacle of the crowd, they found an original way to place the crippled before Jesus by stripping the roof over the place where Jesus was (ἀπεστέγασαν τὴν στέγην ὅπου ἦν Mark 2:4), since they were unwilling to give up until they brought the one in need close to Lord. At this moment Jesus saw the men's faith (ἰδὼν ὁ Ἰησοῦς τὴν πίστιν αὐτῶν Mark 2:5) as only God can see what is hidden from the corporeal eye. The text never says that Jesus' sees the faith of the paralytic. The only object of Jesus' seeing is "their faith" (τὴν πίστιν αὐτῶν), i.e. the faith of the four litter-bearers that sets in motion the act of divine healing. The verb employed to describe the seeing of Jesus is ὁράω in its aorist

15 Cf. Walter Grundmann, *Das Evangelium nach Markus*. THNT 2 (Berlin: Evangelische Verlagsanstalt, 1977), 283; John Donahue and Daniel Harrington, *The Gospel of Mark* (Collegeville, MN: Liturgical Press, 2007), 303.

participle: ἰδὼν which can be interpreted as a completed action that is not prolonged in time but is relative in the temporal sequence, indicating a logical succession of actions that culminates with physical and spiritual healing,[16] e.g. "and Jesus, after seeing their faith, says to the paralytic (καὶ ἰδὼν ὁ Ἰησοῦς τὴν πίστιν αὐτῶν λέγει τῷ παραλυτικῷ)" (Mark 2:5). Therefore after Jesus sees the nameless men putting the paralytic in front of him, what comes as a consequence is "the healing of body and soul conjointly."[17]

The explicit object of Jesus' seeing is the "faith" (τὴν πίστιν Mark 2:5) of the anonymous bearers which can be demonstrated with actions. In this case their faith is not just seen in the outward manifestations, as evidenced by in their creative way of surpassing several obstacles, but the text indicates that Jesus literally can see the inner spiritual sphere of the soul of each of the unnamed men.

The grammatical sequence of the lexemes demonstrates the theology of the statement affirmed: καὶ ἰδὼν ὁ Ἰησοῦς τὴν πίστιν αὐτῶν (Mark 2:5). The syntactic structure of the proposition, conjunction + verb (participle) + subject + object (accusative), reveals the direct connection between the subject, Jesus, who is seeing the only object of his particular visual perception, which in this case is "the faith of them" (τὴν πίστιν αὐτῶν). The text never places these nameless men as the direct objects, in the accusative, of the seeing of Jesus, which means that in this specific context the distinct personhood of each unnamed man fades into the background of the narrative while their faith, as the focal point of the attention of Jesus, is brought into the foreground of the narrative. The reader can perceive in Mark's account that Jesus' seeing is unfailingly metaphysical, distinguishing itself from any kind of human visual perception.

The passage of Mark 5:31-32 provides additional evidence for the contrast between Jesus' seeing and his disciples' visual perception. The passage is framed in the healing context of a woman with hemorrhages (Mark 5:25-34), which is a narrative inserted in the story regarding the raising of Jairus' daughter (5:21-24.35-43). This literary device, commonly called the *Markan sandwich*, is not unfamiliar to the Markan narrative, presenting itself as a personal characteristic of the author's style, as can be seen in 3:20-35; 11:12-25; 14:53-72.

The context depicts a woman who had been suffering from continuous hemorrhages for twelve years (γυνὴ οὖσα ἐν ῥύσει αἵματος δώδεκα ἔτη Mark 5:25). This unnamed woman knew the Lord was passing by and used this opportunity to touch at least a piece of his cloak in order to be healed: ἔλεγεν γὰρ ὅτι ἐὰν ἅψωμαι κἂν τῶν ἱματίων αὐτοῦ σωθήσομαι (Mark 5:28). When she did, Jesus

16 Cf. Maximilian Zerwick, *Biblical Greek* (Roma: Pontificium Istitutum Biblicum, 2001) n. 268; Guerra-Gómez, *El idioma*, 298.

17 Clement of Alexandria, "Christ the Educator 1.4," in *Ante-Nicene Fathers*, eds. A. Roberts, J. Donaldson, and A. C. Coxe (Peabody, MA: Hendrickson, 1994), II, 2.

realized what had happened, and when asking his disciples "who touched him" (Τίς μου ἥψατο τῶν ἱματίων; Mark 5:30b), they did not understand why he asked because the crowd was pressing on him: καὶ ἔλεγον αὐτῷ οἱ μαθηταὶ αὐτοῦ· βλέπεις τὸν ὄχλον συνθλίβοντά σε καὶ λέγεις· τίς μου ἥψατο; (Mark 5:31).

Responding to Jesus' question, the disciples employed the verb βλέπω in present indicative to describe their perception of the event: "You see (Βλέπεις) the multitude pressing in on you." The disciples' notion of an external (physical) seeing is made manifest by their statement. They are not yet capable of going beyond what is physically apparent or evident, which also indicates the increasing level of misunderstanding in their relationship with Jesus.[18] A sharp contrast is provided by the Markan narrative through the emphatic verbal construction employed to portray Jesus' seeing of the same reality.

In the passage of Mark 5:32, Jesus' seeing is indicated with two verbs of visual perception: περιεβλέπετο ἰδεῖν. One is the conjugated verb περιεβλέπετο in its imperfect indicative form, which connotes a durative action taking place, meaning that Jesus' vision was ongoing (progressive verbal aspect), not only occurring at this particular time: "he was looking around."[19] Regarding this translation, there is a discrepancy between the Greek text of Nestle–Aland and the *lectiones* of KJV, NAB, NAS[20] among others, that present: "he looked around." The English renditions indicate an aorist indicative, while the Greek text presents an imperfect indicative. The second verb of visual perception used in the Markan dual construction is presented in active aorist infinitive of ὁράω, ἰδεῖν which points towards the finality of the action, taking place at a particular time. The verb itself, ἰδεῖν, bears with it the semantic connotation of individualizing somebody by means of an intense visual observation.[21] Consequently Jesus' seeing is hardly a superficial glance at the crowd. Rather, it is a selective and personal seeing seeking to identify the concrete person in her whole existential complexity.

The seeing of the Lord is effective because it provokes a succession of events, starting with the self-identification of the woman (5:33) that ultimately produces a complete spiritual healing that gives birth to the faith in Jesus as the Messiah and Son of God (5:34). In this line of thought the words of Ephrem the Syrian (306–373 CE) are appropriate:

---

18 Cf. Marie-Joseph Lagrange, *Évangile selon St. Marc* (Paris: J. Gabalda, 1966), 141.

19 Cf. Zerwick, *Biblical Greek*, n. 241; Vincenzo Scippa, "Stile e spunti di teologia in Mc 5,21-43," *Asprenas* 30 (1983): 224.

20 KJV: King James Version (1611, 1769); NAB: New American Bible (1970, 1986, 1991, 2010); NAS: New American Standard Bible (1977).

21 Cf. Juan Mateos and Fernando Camacho, *Il Vangelo di Marco. Analisi linguistica e commento esegetico* (Assisi: Cittadella Editrice, 1997), I, 457.

> Glory to you, hidden Son of God, because your healing power is proclaimed through the hidden suffering of the afflicted woman. Through this woman whom they could see, the witnesses were enabled to behold the divinity that cannot be seen. Through the Son's own healing power His divinity became known. Through the afflicted woman's being healed her faith was made manifest. She caused Him to be proclaimed, and indeed was honored with Him. For truth was being proclaimed together with its heralds. If she was a witness to His divinity, He in turn was a witness to her faith ... He saw through to her hidden faith, and gave her a visible healing.[22]

4. Contemplation

The scene of the poor and generous widow in Mark 12:41-44 has the narrative function of portraying an incisive dissimilarity with the self-promoted scribes who are heavily criticized by Jesus in the immediate context of Mark 12:38-40. This episode is worth mentioning in relation to the present topic because it shows one of the two occurrences in Mark's Gospel of the verb θεωρέω taking Jesus as its subject. The other instance is Mark 5:38, which narrates the raising of the daughter of Jairus. The pericope states that on arriving at the official's house, Jesus observes/contemplates (θεωρεῖ) the commotion of the people. His contemplation penetrates funeral laments taking place in the narrative that function as proof of the fatality of death. Nevertheless, perception of her death is not the end but an opportunity for a new gift of life that comes from God.[23]

Concerning the poor widow's episode, Mark sets the narrative in the Second Temple, which had eight gates within its enclosure: two on the South, four on the West, one on the North, and one on the East. The enclosed space was divided into several courts. The largest one was the court of the Gentiles, to which everyone had access; it was separated from the other spaces by a balustrade prohibiting the Gentiles from passing into the other courts. After the court of the Gentiles comes the court of the women which was five steps above the court of the Gentiles, and the women could not pass beyond this area.[24] The next cloister was

---

22 Ephrem the Syrian, "Commentary on Tatian's Diatessaron," Leloir 1990:88; JSSS 2:129, in *Mark. ACCS NT II*, eds. Oden and Hall, II, 70.

23 Cf. Rudolf Pesch, *Il vangelo di Marco*: *Parte prima. Testo greco e traduzione ai cappitoli 1,1 - 8,26* (Brescia: Paideia, 1980), I, 486-487.

24 "The cloisters [of the outmost court] were in breadth thirty cubits, while the entire compass of it was by measure six furlongs, including the tower of Antonia; those entire courts that were exposed to the air were laid with stones of all sorts. When you go through these [first] cloisters, unto the second [court of the] temple, there was a partition made of stone all round, whose height was three cubits: its construction was very elegant; upon it stood pillars, at equal distances from one another, declaring the law of purity, some in Greek, and some in Roman letters, that 'no foreigner should go within that

of the court of Israel, or the court of the men, followed by the court of the priests, and finally the Holy of Holies or Sanctus Sanctorum.[25] Jesus was sitting against one of the thirteen treasury boxes (γαζοφυλάκιον), contemplating (ἐθεώρει) everyone who was giving their offering. It is crucial to highlight the tense of the verb θεωρέω, which is in its imperfect indicative form, ἐθεώρει. The use of the imperfect indicative describes an action in progress that began in the past and is not yet finalized or concluded,[26] so ἐθεώρει is properly translated as "Jesus was contemplating." The Greek text clearly presents the verb in the imperfect indicative, signifying an action in progress as does the Vulgata: "sedens Iesus contra gazofilacium *aspiciebat* (was seeing) quomodo turba iactaret aes in gazofilacium" (12:41). It would be inaccurate to translate ἐθεώρει as "he beheld" (ASV, DRA, ETH, GNV, KJV),[27] or "he observed" (NAB, NJB, ESV, CJB),[28]

---

sanctuary' for that second [court of the] temple was called 'the Sanctuary,' and was ascended to by fourteen steps from the first court. This court was four-square, and had a wall about it peculiar to itself; the height of its buildings, although it were on the outside forty cubits, was hidden by the steps, and on the inside that height was but twenty-five cubits; for it being built over against a higher part of the hill with steps, it was no further to be entirely discerned within, being covered by the hill itself. Beyond these thirteen steps there was the distance of ten cubits; this was all plain; whence there were other steps, each of five cubits a-piece, that led to the gates, which gates on the north and south sides were eight, on each of those sides four, and of necessity two on the east. For since there was a partition built for the women on that side, as the proper place wherein they were to worship, there was a necessity for a second gate for them: this gate was cut out of its wall, over against the first gate. There was also on the other sides one southern and one northern gate, through which was a passage into the court of the women; for as to the other gates, the women were not allowed to pass through them; nor when they went through their own gate could they go beyond their own wall. This place was allotted to the women of our own country, and of other countries, provided they were of the same nation, and that equally. The western part of this court had no gate at all, but the wall was built entirely on that side. But then the cloisters which were betwixt the gates extended from the wall inward, before the chambers; for they were supported by very fine and large pillars. These cloisters were single, and, excepting their magnitude, were no way inferior to those of the lower court." Flavius Josephus, *Jewish War* 5.5.2, in *The Genuine Works of Flavius Josephus, the Jewish Historian*, trans. William Whiston (Boston 1737) accessed October 17, 2013, http: // www.ccel.org / ccel / josephus / complete. iii. vi.v. html.

25 Cf. John McKenzie, "Temple," *DB*, 875-876.

26 Cf. Daniel Wallace, *Greek Grammar beyond the Basis. An exegetical Syntax of the New Testament* (Grand Rapids: Zondervan Publishing House 1996), 541.543; Blass-Debrunner: n. 325.327

27 ASV: American Standard Version (1901); DRA: Douay-Rheims 1899 American Edition; ETH: Etheridge Translation of the NT Peshitta (1849); GNV: Geneva Bible (1599); KJV: King James Version (1611, 1769).

given that the aforementioned translations would be the proper rendering of the aorist form of θεωρέω, and that form does not exist in the *textus receptus* of Nestle–Aland.

What does Jesus see? The object of the visual perception is the manner, the *modus* (πῶς / *quomodo*), in which the people are depositing their offering. According to the Mishnah Shekalim 6:5, in the temple there were "thirteen chests" (γαζοφυλάκιον) in the form of trumpets upon which were inscriptions specifying the purpose of the offering. The treasury box or *gazophylákion* (γαζοφυλάκιον) refers to the receptacle in the Court of Women used to collect freewill offerings as attested by Flavius Josephus in *Jewish War* 6.5.2 (6.282).[29] Jesus contemplates with the eyes of God, a divine capability that allows him to perceive not the quantity of money but the intention behind the offering. Jesus was recognizing the genuine sacrifice hidden beneath the two lepta or small copper coins of the widow, which were the smallest and least valuable coins in circulation in Palestine, worth one-half of "quadrans" (in Greek κοδράντης) or 1/128 of a "denarius", which would be a day's salary for a common laborer.[30] The metaphysical or spiritual seeing of the Lord is confirmed in the instructions imparted to his disciples in vv. 43-44:

> And calling his disciples, (he) said to them, "Amen I say unto you, that this poor widow threw in more than all the others who were throwing in to the treasury, because all of them threw in of their abundance, but she from her poverty threw in everything she had, even all her living.[31]

---

28 NAB: New American Bible (1970, 1986, 1991, 2010); NJB: New Jerusalem Bible (1985); ESV: English Standard Version (2001, 2007, 2011); CJB: Complete Jewish Bible (1998).

29 "And now the Romans, judging that it was in vain to spare what was round about the holy house, burnt all those places, as also the remains of the cloisters and the gates, two excepted; the one on the east side, and the other on the south; both which, however, they burnt afterward. They also burnt down the treasury chambers, in which was an immense quantity of money, and an immense number of garments, and other precious goods there reposited; and, to speak all in a few words, there it was that the entire riches of the Jews were heaped up together, while the rich people had there built themselves chambers [to contain such furniture]. The soldiers also came to the rest of the cloisters that were in the outer [court of the] temple, whither the women and children, and a great mixed multitude of the people, fled, in number about six thousand." Flavius Josephus, *Jewish War* 6.5.2, trans. William Whiston, accessed October 17, 2013, http: // www.ccel.org/ ccel/ josephus/ complete.iii.vii.v.html.

30 Cf. Rudolf Schnackenburg, *Vangelo secondo Marco* (Roma: Città Nuova Editrice, 2002) 335-336; Donahue and Harrington, *Mark*, 364-365.

31 Author's translation.

Using an emphatic "amen" (ἀμὴν), Jesus assures his disciples that the underprivileged widow put in more (πλεῖον Mark 12:43) than all the other contributors to the treasury, and the reason for such an affirmation is based upon his spiritual and personal observation of the widow who put in everything that she had, meaning her entire wealth and way of living (ὅλον τὸν βίον αὐτῆς Mk 12:44). The widow's total self-giving to God cannot go unperceived by the one who sees everything. The Lord sees what is lacking in those who apparently give much more money from what abounded to them, and what is rich in the heart of a poor nameless widow.

5. Note of Conclusion

As a précis of the Markan characteristics of Jesus' seeing, it is possible to highlight the following considerations:

The initiative of seeing comes from Jesus, especially in the pericope of *sequela*. Jesus' seeing, as mentioned previously, remains the first step of the vocation, being the primary phase of selection that motivates the calling.[32] This phenomenon is uncommon in the Semitic mindset, since typically it was the disciple who aspired to be accepted by a particular Rabbi or rabbinic school of the time. The summoning of the disciples marks an original and creative initiative of Jesus that is performed with a kind of discontinuity with his culture.[33] At this point, it is convenient to allude to Karl Barth, who, making a paraphrase of the famous Cartesian expression *Cogito ergo sum*, affirms *Cogitor ergo sum*, meaning that in the moment that *I am* thought or perceived by God, in that instant *I exist*, *I am*. The pasivus theologicus in the latter affirmation expresses the initiative that belongs to the divinity who always wants to reach out to a person out of love and kindness.[34]

Jesus' seeing is intuitive and personal. He sees the totality of a person scrutinizing every aspect of their spiritual essence. The direct objects of the seeing of Jesus are the divine reality of the situation, the faith of the person seen, the interior of a person, and his or her spiritual state. His sight captures everything that is hidden to an ordinary human eye. His seeing extends beyond the physical limitations, penetrating earthly masks and seeing the spiritual or supernatural dimension. This also highlights how his seeing is not casual. It has authority and

32 Cf. Joel Marcus, *Mark 1-8*, AncB 27A (New York – London: Doubleday, 2000), 183.

33 Cf. Karl H. Rengstorf, "μαθητής," *TDNT* IV, 446-447; Martin Hengel, *The Charismatic Leader and His Followers*, trans. J. Greig, SNTW (Edinburgh: T&T Clark, 1981), 50-51; James R. Edwards, *The Gospel according to Mark* (Grand Rapids: Eerdmans, 2002), 49.

34 Cf. J. Palachuvattil, *"He saw,"* 101. n.19.

purpose in the dynamic behavior of Jesus; it is the preamble that initiates a calling, act of mercy, teaching, miracle, exorcism or healing. Therefore his seeing is *effective*, which means that the action immediately following after his special perception is already contained in his seeing, e.g., the passages of vocation: Mark 1:16-20; 2:14.[35] Thus, it is possible to conclude that Jesus' visual perception in Mark's Gospel is more than human, and that it equates to the supernatural seeing of God.

35 Cf. Palachuvattil, *"He saw,"* 102; Edwards, *Mark*, 49-50.81-82.

Chapter VII

The Seeing of the Demons

1. The Pericopes

In the New Testament demons are presented as real beings (Matt 4,1.17; 8,29; 12,43; Mark 1,34; Luke 4,33-36; 8,31; John 12,31; 13,2.31; 14,17). They are entities opposing the action of God, wanting to destroy the economy of salvation. The demons influence and manipulate the body and soul of a person (a demoniac), inflicting a variety of physical manifestations that can be perceived, according to the viewpoint of someone immersed in the Semitic mindset, as illness or infirmities, such as dumbness (Matt 9:32), blindness (Matt 12:22), epilepsy (Mark 9:17-27), and insanity (Mark 5:1-5). Conversely, it is possible to perceive in Mark's Gospel the differentiation between demoniacs and those who are afflicted with ordinary bodily maladies, i.e., Mark 1:32 16:17.18.[1]

In our study of visual perception in Mark's narrative, it is crucial for us to focus our attention on three important passages that summarize the consistent behavioral pattern of the demons. As illustrative examples, these passages show us the special characteristics of the manner of their "seeing" in the specific contexts of possessions and exorcisms. These essential texts, in their Greek version, are presented with the principal verbs of perception in italic in order to show their usage by the author.

Mark 3:11-12: καὶ τὰ πνεύματα τὰ ἀκάθαρτα, ὅταν αὐτὸν *ἐθεώρουν*, προσέπιπτον αὐτῷ καὶ ἔκραζον λέγοντες ὅτι σὺ εἶ ὁ υἱὸς τοῦ θεοῦ. καὶ πολλὰ ἐπετίμα αὐτοῖς ἵνα μὴ αὐτὸν φανερὸν ποιήσωσιν.

---

1 Cf. Werner Foerster, "δαίμων," *TDNT* II, 18-19; Gregory E. Sterling, "Jesus as Exorcist: An Analysis of Matthew 17:14-20; Mark 9:14-29; Luke 9:37-43a," *CBQ* 55 (1993): 477; Edwards, *Mark*, 277-278.

Mark 5:6-7: καὶ *ἰδὼν* τὸν Ἰησοῦν ἀπὸ μακρόθεν ἔδραμεν καὶ προσεκύνησεν αὐτῷ καὶ κράξας φωνῇ μεγάλῃ λέγει· τί ἐμοὶ καὶ σοί, Ἰησοῦ υἱὲ τοῦ θεοῦ τοῦ ὑψίστου; ὁρκίζω σε τὸν θεόν, μή με βασανίσῃς.

Mark 9:20: καὶ ἤνεγκαν αὐτὸν πρὸς αὐτόν. καὶ *ἰδὼν* αὐτὸν τὸ πνεῦμα εὐθὺς συνεσπάραξεν αὐτόν, καὶ πεσὼν ἐπὶ τῆς γῆς ἐκυλίετο ἀφρίζων.

The immediate context of the passage of Mark 3:11-12 is the pericope of Mark 3:7-12. This section is actually the longest summary in the Markan Gospel. Following the opinion of R. T. France regarding the *Redaktionskritic*, the text of Mark 3:7-12 stands on its own as a self-contained unit summarizing the healing activity of Jesus.[2] The unit, therefore, could be inserted at almost any point in Jesus' ministry in Galilee, functioning as a narrative bridge that concludes one narrative section but at the same time introduces the section that follows. But why did the real author of Mark's Gospel insert the pericope in the actual position of the Gospel that corresponds to 3:7-12, namely, its final canonical redaction? Possible answers to this question can be summarized in three ideas.

a) The real author of Mark wanted to emphasize the popularity of Jesus due to his divine power and authority. It is crucial for the author of the Gospel of Mark to demonstrate the success of Jesus in Galilee from the beginning of his public ministry in the region.

b) The Markan summary helps to understand the overall intention of the author who prersents in his Gospel the sharp contrast between the success of Jesus in Galilee and the hardship and lack of acceptance of his ministry in Jerusalem. In this manner both geographical contexts embody two theological standpoints that represent antagonistic reactions in front of Jesus' message and deeds. Galilee embodies the positive acceptance of Jesus while Jerusalem the rejection that leads to the killing of Jesus.[3] Therefore, Galilee remains in the Markan Theology as the privileged field of action for Jesus in his salutary ministry, that is why the author presents him as a teacher, healer, and exorcist in front of a multitude of followers who also serve as witnesses of the veracity of his words and deeds.[4]

2 Cf. France, *The Gospel of Mark*, 152.

3 Cf. M. Völkel, "Γαλιλαία," *DENT*, I, 701; Bas van Iersel, *Marco. La Lettura e la Risposta. Un Commento* (Brescia: Queriniana, 2000), 66-68.

4 Cf. Dempsey Rosales-Acosta, *La victoria sobre el poder de la muerte. Ensayo semántico y narrativo del texto griego de Marcos 9:30-32*. Series Investigación (Sevilla: Círculo Rojo, 2012) 67-68.

c) The great multitude (πολὺ πλῆθος Mark 3:7.8)—larger group of enthusiasts who witness Jesus' miracles by bringing to him the sick, suffering, and demoniacs—serves as a contrast to stress the selection of the twelve, the inner group of followers who are portrayed as special companions of the Lord.[5] The main interest of the large multitude is the physical and spiritual healing or deliverance effected by the power of Jesus. For this reason people came from far afield to follow him. This persistent and demanding attitude of the people described by the Markan author continues throughout the ministry of Jesus to such a degree that the Markan author feels compelled to note that Jesus must actively seek moments of solitude. "They have not come out of pure disinterested concern to hear the message of the kingdom of God, but to witness and to benefit from his power in healing (v. 10) and exorcism (v.11-12)."[6]

The verse of Mark 3:10 talks about the diseases (μάστιγας) that afflicted many (πολλοὺς) and their respective healings (ἐθεράπευσεν) that restore wholeness of life to those who were suffering. The verse functions as an anaphoric reference that sends the reader to a previous section, since this portrait of physical healing has been presented already in Mark 1:34, which also summarizes Jesus' exorcisms. It is significant to note that Mark 3:11 treats the demonic possessions as something different from sickness or maladies. Starting from verses 11-12 the exorcism context narrates the encounter of Jesus with the passive hosts of the impure spirits (τὰ πνεύματα τὰ ἀκάθαρτα). The voices of the possessed human is used to profess or cry out (ἔκραζον λέγοντες) Christological statements, submission, and possible negotiations with the highest power while their human bodies are utilized by the τὰ πνεύματα τὰ ἀκάθαρτα as the physical human instrument of interrelationship with the social reality and also to express submission (προσέπιπτον).

The text of Mark 3:11-12 can be classified as one summary inserted into a larger Markan summary (Mark 3:7-12). This inner summary concentrates a prolonged period of time into two verses in which the characters, "the unclean spirits" (τὰ πνεύματα τὰ ἀκάθαρτα), meaning that the people the unclean spirits possess and through whom they speak were beholding or contemplating (ἐθεώρουν) Jesus repeatedly on different occasions. The use of the verb θεωρέω in third person plural imperfect indicative, ἐθεώρουν, indicates a regularly recurring activity in past time that can be classified as habitual.[7] Most of the English versions translate the verb taking the verbal aspect into account, rendering the Greek verb as an aorist, which translates as "beheld" or "saw", accompanied with the adverb

5 Cf. France, *The Gospel of Mark*, 153; Leander E. Keck, "Mark 3:7-12 and Mark's Christology," *JBL* 84, no. 4 (1965): 342-345.

6 France, *The Gospel of Mark*, 153.

7 Cf. Wallace, *Greek Grammar*, 548; Blass-Debrunner, n. 325.327.

of time "whenever" or "when," in order to express the habitual character of the imperfect. Therefore the summary passage contains a pattern of behavior that can be described as a spiritual perception typical of supernatural beings. Such a way of seeing is implicit in every encounter of a demoniac with Jesus narrated in Mark's Gospel.

The verses of Mark 5:6-7 are inserted in the episode commonly known as the exorcism of the Gerasene Demoniac (Mark 5:1-20). The episode stresses the power and authority of Jesus that can control the untamable dark forces present not only in one demon at a time but in a large multitude of them, for in this passage the demons are a "legion" cohabiting in the body of one man: λεγιὼν ὄνομά μοι, ὅτι πολλοί ἐσμεν (Mark 5:9).

The episode also has an anaphoric and proleptic function. One of the most significant components of Jesus' ministry in Galilee consists in the exorcisms as described in this section and two other important Markan summaries, 1:32-34 and 3:11-12. However, this passage silmultaneously prepares the readers for subsequent action coming in the narrative, especially Mark 6:7.13, 7:24-30, and 9:14-29.

The exorcism in Mark 5:1-20 is one of the most spectacular in the narrative because of its distinctive features, including: the geographical context, which is a Gentile territory, the portrait of the demoniac condition (5:2-5), the number of the demons or impure spirits possessing the person, their acknowledgment of the Christological identity, their name, their request, their expulsion from the host and the possession of the pigs, the destruction of the pigs, and the full spiritual, physical, and psychological healing of the one who was possessed.

The interest of the real author of Mark in this particular episode becomes evident in the analysis of the synoptic statistic of the Greek words used in the pericope of Mark and Matthew. The word count of Mark's pericope is a total of 330 lexemes while the length of the story in Matthew embodies a total of 135 lexemes.[8] Hence Matthew uses less than 50% of the words used by Mark to describe the same event, making this one of the unique cases in which Mark has a lectio longior in comparison with Matthew, who in this case presents the lectio brevior.[9] The special attention dedicated by the Markan author to this event serves to underline forcefully the Christological authority explicitly expressed in the spiritual realm and implicitly communicated through the Gentile spectators who were afraid and disturbed by Jesus' presence in their midst. The details that the Markan author includes in this particular expulsion story highlight an im-

8 Cf. France, *The Gospel of Mark*, 226.

9 Mark has 661 verses, Matthew has 1,068 verses, and Luke 1,149. Therefore 80% of Mark is reproduced in Matthew and 65% in Luke. Cf. Frans Neirynck, "Synoptic Problem," *NJBC*, 588.

portant theme present in the ministry of the Jewish Messiah. The Christological mission is described in the Markan theology as a message that surpasses the boundaries of Israel in order to reach those who traditionally are classified as outsiders and incapable of receiving of God's blessings.

The verse of Mark 9:20 is part of other episode of exorcism that corresponds to the pericope of Mark 9:14-29, which is commonly known as the healing of a possessed boy. The beginning and the end of the episode (9:14-29) indicates a thematic *inclusio* that demonstrates the failure of the disciples in the dealings with the demons. As a general narrative schema I propose the following concentric structure[10] that conveys the aforementioned ideas:

a. The failure of the disciples: 9:14-19
    b. The encounter between Jesus and demoniac: 9:20-24
    b'. Exorcism and restoration to health: 9:25-27
a'. Disciples' reaction, reason of their failure: 9:28-29

The incapacity of the disciples concerning the expulsion of demons stresses the divine ἐξουσία of Jesus. The center of the story focuses on the encounter of the possessed boy and Jesus that produces violent effects (9:20). The outcome of the encounter is the boy's total restoration to health. The theme of the divine authority of Jesus is intertwined with the notion of the incredulity of Jesus' generation, including his disciples and the father of the possessed boy (γενεὰ ἄπιστος Mark 9:19). The victory over the power of the demons, who felt compelled to inquire into the reason of their failure (9:28-29), makes the contrast between Jesus and his disciples, who progressively distance themselves from their master, even more obvious.[11]

The pericopes of Mark 5:6 and 9:20 present the verb ὁράω as a nominative masculine participle in singular active aorist: ἰδὼν. In Greek, participles can function in a sentence as an adjective and have morphological variations similar to the declensions of adjectives. Unlike other adjectives, though, a participle is formed from a verb, and like verbs, a participle has a subject and an object, assuming the modifications and the verbal aspects of the Greek tenses.[12] For this

10 Cf. Rosales-Acosta, *La victoria sobre el poder de la muerte*, 133. See also different concentric structures in Friedrich G. Lang, "Sola Gratia im Markusevangelium: Die Soteriologie des Markus nach 9,14-29 und 10,17-31," in *Rechtfertigung: Festschrift für Ernst Käsemann zum 70 Geburtstag*, eds. Johannes Friedrich, Wolfgang Pöhlmann, and Peter Stuhlmacher (Tübingen: J. C. B. Mohr Vandenhoeck und Ruprecht, 1976), 322; Sharyn Dowd, *Reading Mark. A Literary and Theological Commentary on the Second Gospel* (Macon, GA: Smyth & Helwys, 2000), 94.

11 Cf. Rosales-Acosta, *La victoria sobre el poder de la muerte*, 132-133.

12 Cf. Guerra-Gómez, *El Idioma*, 297-298.

reason the term participle derives from the Latin *participare*, "to participate," because its nature consists in its participation of the essential aspects of the adjective and a verb. The participle expresses a secondary action in the narrative, an action subordinated to a principal verb. Because ἰδὼν is an aorist participle in Mark 5:6 and 9:20, it denotes a single, succinct action, not durative in time. The verbal sequence manifested in the participle aorist expresses anteriority, thus portraying a relation of logical succession of cause and effect, which is why the majority of the English versions translate the participle in these pericopes as "saw."[13] The participle in Mark 5:6 and 9:20, behaves more like a verb, having a subject, the demons, and an object of observation, who, in this case, is the person of Jesus. In both cases the demons first "saw" (ἰδὼν) Jesus, and they then reacted according to what they saw. The seeing of the demoniacs becomes the first step from which subsequent demoniac reactions emerge in violent manifestations as expressed in the episodes of Mark 5:7 and 9:20.26.

2. Behavioral Pattern of the Demoniacs

A parallel reading of the three texts mentioned above enables the reader to determine the following pattern of conduct of the unclean spirits:

a) In each narrative the narrator describes an encounter between Jesus and a demoniac or demons, and in such cases the initiative of the visual perception belongs to the unclean spirit. In Mark's narrative, the first awareness of the unnoticeable divinity of Jesus always comes from the spiritual entity acting against the salutary economy of the incarnated Logos: 3:11; 5:6 and 9:20. The demons are the subject of the verb that communicates a habitual action (3:11) or a precise perception that precedes the reactions that is motivated by their seeing (5:6; 9:20).

b) The direct object of the seeing of the demons is Jesus, so their vision is a Christological experience. They identify him immediately, and in doing so, the narrator vividly describes their reaction: "they would fall down (προσέπιπτον) before him and cry out (ἔκραζον)" (Mark 3:11) and in Mark 5:6 the voice of the narrator says: "and seeing Jesus from a distance (καὶ ἰδὼν τὸν Ἰησοῦν ἀπὸ μακρόθεν), he ran and *fell on his knees / prostrated himself* (προσεκύνησεν) in front of him."[14] The verb προσπίπτω in Mark 3:11 indicates a physical response of reverence and respect to a higher power, carrying more of a connotation of

13 Cf. Blass-Debrunner, n. 339. For the argumentation regarding the verbal aspect of the participle aorist, see Zerwick, *Biblical Greek*, nn. 261-265.

14 Possible options of translation proposed by the author.

submission than worship or homage. The verb is used in the imperfect tense, προσέπιπτον, which denotes a repeated or habitual action of submission rather than a single act of worship or homage.[15] In the episode of Mark 5:6, the verb προσκυνέω is used in the third person singular aorist active indicative, προσεκύνησεν, which marks a particular instance of submission, indicating a physical reaction of reverence and respect to a higher power.[16] These passages therefore connote an image of prostration before a superior authority that can be illustrated in other texts such as Gen 17:3; Dan 3:5; Matt 2:11; 4:9. Mark's author, in speaking of the agency of the demons rather than the victim, states that they never run away from the presence of Jesus. This is an unexpected characteristic of the demons in the narrative, since it is easier to imagine that they would flee from the perturbing and dominant presence of Jesus. The Gospel, however, is clear with respect to this aspect: the demons stay and prostrate, dually indicating that there is no escape from the presence of God and that his absolute power is capable of overcoming them.[17]

c) The demoniac proclamations are Christological statements. The demons usually have the capacity to speak by themselves or in their own name through the possessed persons (Mark 1:23-24; 5:7; also see Matt 8:29). However, when they prostate themselves before Jesus, their deed is complemented with a profession of faith that reveals the true nature of their seeing: "you are the Son of God (Σὺ εἶ ὁ υἱὸς τοῦ θεοῦ)" (Mark 3:11[b]) or "Jesus, Son of the Most High God (Ἰησοῦ υἱὲ τοῦ θεοῦ τοῦ ὑψίστου;)" (Mark 5:7; also 1:24).

This ultimate truth about Jesus reveals an explicit Christological confession, already announced by God in Mark 1:11: Σὺ εἶ ὁ υἱός μου ὁ ἀγαπητός and 9:7, Οὗτός ἐστιν ὁ υἱός μου ὁ ἀγαπητός. Although it is proclaimed now through human lips by a supernatural entity, the divine identity still remains hidden from the general public.[18] Such a statement demonstrates that the demons can also observe what is underneath the different layers of human appearances, being able to see without difficulty what others could not see, namely, Jesus' divine nature.

d) As representatives of a supernatural dimension, the demons possess a knowledge and visual perception superior to that of the disciples, followers or

15 Cf. Ezra Gould, *Critical and Exegetical Commentary on the Gospel according to St. Mark*. ICC (Edinburgh: T&T Clark, 1961), 56; M. Eugene Boring, *Mark. A Commentary* (NTL; Louisville: Westminster John Knox Press, 2006), 98-99.

16 Cf. Bas van Iersel, *Mark. A Reader-Response Commentary* (London, UK – New York, NY: T&T Clark, 1998), 198.

17 Cf. Marcus, *Mark 1-8*, 259.

18 Cf. France, *The Gospel of Mark*, 155.

any other human in Mark's narrative. There is therefore a profound irony in the Gospel narratives when the reader notices that the ones whom Jesus came to combat are the first to recognize him for what he truly is; on the other hand, the irony of the narrative becomes more evident in the superficial seeing of the scribes who affirm that Jesus is possessed by Beelzebub and is driving out demons by the prince of the demons (Mark 3:22). The statement of the scribes declares a theological notion that opposes the Christological confession proclaimed by the demons. While the demoniacs affirm that Jesus is the Son of God (Mark 3:11[b] Σὺ εἶ ὁ υἱὸς τοῦ θεοῦ) or the Son of the most high God (Mark 5:7: Ἰησοῦ υἱὲ τοῦ θεοῦ τοῦ ὑψίστου), the scribes profess an anti-Christological assertion. For them Beelzebul is contained in the person of Jesus: "he has Beelzebul" (Βεελζεβοὺλ ἔχει Mark 3:22).

The statement of the scribes is antagonistic to the declaration of the incarnation of the Logos in the person of Jesus (Jn 1:1.14), and in this manner they communicate a line of thought that contradicts the divine logic of the salutary economy of the Trinitarian God. So for the scribes it is not the Logos who is incarnate in Jesus but Beelzebul himself. It is not the Father who perfoms wonderful deeds in the Son, but Beelzebul who acts in the person of Jesus driving out other demons: ὅτι ἐν τῷ ἄρχοντι τῶν δαιμονίων ἐκβάλλει τὰ δαιμόνια (Mark 3:22). The attitude of the scribes in Mark's Gospel exemplifies the theological affirmation of the author of John's Gospel when he declares: "He was in the world, and the world was made through him, and the world didn't recognize him. He came to his own, and those who were his own didn't receive him" (Jn 1:10-11). The scribes' declaration demonstrates a physical and superficial perception that leads them to arrive at the erroneous conclusion regarding the identity of Jesus. On the other hand, it is significant to note that the demonic confession of the Christological identity of Jesus indicates a simple proclamation of the truth of his eschatological lordship that does not imply embracing faith, love, and trust in Jesus.[19]

e) Violent reactions are distinctive behavioral indicators of the demons and of the overwhelming power emanating from Jesus that torments the unclean spirits. The acknowledgment of Jesus' divine nature is expressed with a loud scream (κράξας a participle aorist from the verb κράζω) in Mark 5:7, heightening the theme of pain, which echoes the exorcisms of the demoniac of Capernaum (see Mark 1:21-28). The evil entities inflict pain and suffering on their victims in order to channel their distress and pain produced by the presence of God, as in the case of Mark 9:20, where the wordless reaction of the demon still expresses

---

19 Cf. Ben Witherington III, *The Gospel of Mark. A Socio-Rhetorical Commentary* (Grand Rapids: Eerdmans, 2001), 144; Marcus, *Mark 1-8*, 259.

its vehement response to Jesus: "the spirit immediately tore him (συνεσπάραξεν); and falling upon the earth he rolled foaming." The dramatic suffering inflicted to the possessed person is described with the verb συσπαράσσω which evokes the image of a dog tearing up a carcass. In this particular text, it is used analogically to indicate a convulsion.[20] The violent reactions continue while Jesus is present until he commands the unclean spirit to leave the boy in Mark 9:26.

f) Liberation and total healing are the consequences of the Christological authority in the context of exorcisms. At the end of each encounter between the unclean spirits and Jesus, the outcome is a liberating experience for the possessed person that involves a restoration of the wholeness that was lost because of the evil presence. The completeness and totality of the healing provides evidence for the supreme power of Jesus over the demoniac forces, e.g., Mark 9:26-27. His supremacy can be seen overtly in the permission asked by the demons to go into the pigs in Mark 5:12, which was granted by Jesus (5:13), causing the deliverance of the man who had been possessed, and restoring him to his natural condition as a social person capable of leading a harmonious life (5:14-16).

As a consequence of what has been explained above, we can conclude that the demons' seeing is also metaphysical since they are considered spiritual entities who can perceive what is proper of the supernatural realm. Therefore one can readily agree with the words of Athanasius in his work entitled *On the Incarnation of the Word 32.4*: "the spirits especially see through what is unseen by human eyes."[21]

---

20 Cf. France, *The Gospel of Mark*, 366.

21 Oden and Hall, *Mark*, 64.

Chapter VIII

The Visual Perception of the Women: Theōréō

The reader finds in the context of the Crucifixion and the Empty Tomb that the visually perceptive characters are the women (γυναῖκες), especially Mary of Magdala, Mary the mother of James the younger, and Salome. The evangelists describe their action in Mark 15:40-41.47 and 16:4 with the verb θεωρέω, as we can note in the pericopes of the 28th edition of the Nestle–Aland:

Mark 15:40-41: Ἦσαν δὲ καὶ γυναῖκες ἀπὸ μακρόθεν *θεωροῦσαι*, ἐν αἷς καὶ Μαρία ἡ Μαγδαληνὴ καὶ Μαρία ἡ Ἰακώβου τοῦ μικροῦ καὶ Ἰωσῆτος μήτηρ καὶ Σαλώμη, αἳ ὅτε ἦν ἐν τῇ Γαλιλαίᾳ ἠκολούθουν αὐτῷ καὶ διηκόνουν αὐτῷ, καὶ ἄλλαι πολλαὶ αἱ συναναβᾶσαι αὐτῷ εἰς Ἱεροσόλυμα.

Mark 15:47: ἡ δὲ Μαρία ἡ Μαγδαληνὴ καὶ Μαρία ἡ Ἰωσῆτος *ἐθεώρουν* ποῦ τέθειται.

Mark 16:4: καὶ *ἀναβλέψασαι θεωροῦσιν* ὅτι ἀποκεκύλισται ὁ λίθος· ἦν γὰρ μέγας σφόδρα.

What is the meaning of the choice of this particular term in these narratives? The pericopes, in their semantic context, provide a hermeneutic key that the reader can use to identify the nature of the women's perception.

The episode narrated in the passage of Mark 15:40-41 comes immediately after the death of Jesus and the profession of the centurion (15:37-39). The object of the women's perception is Jesus, dead on the Cross. The verb is qualified circumstantially by the expression "from a distance" (ἀπὸ μακρόθεν) which has appeared twice before in the Markan narrative. The first time that it appears it accompanies the verb ὁράω as its circumstantial complement in Mark 5:6[a], where a demoniac is the subject of the visual action: καὶ ἰδὼν τὸν Ἰησοῦν ἀπὸ μακρόθεν, and again in Mark 8:3[b] καί τινες αὐτῶν ἀπὸ μακρόθεν ἥκασιν where

Jesus is the subject of the principal action that leads to the miraculous feeding of the multitude

The passage of Mark 5:6[a] presents a demoniac as the subject implied in the participle of ὁράω: καὶ ἰδὼν τὸν Ἰησοῦν ἀπὸ μακρόθεν ἔδραμεν. The man possessed by the legion, seeing Jesus from a distance, prostates himself before the Lord, and this event produces a series of actions that finishes with the cured man asking to accompany Jesus because he wants to be with him: ἵνα μετ'αὐτοῦ ᾖ (5:18).[1]

The second occasion can be observed in the text of Mark 8:3[b], where Jesus is the subject who performs the principal deeds in the narrative: καί τινες αὐτῶν ἀπὸ μακρόθεν ἥκασιν. The episode describes Jesus, who felt compassion (σπλαγχνίζομαι Mark 8:2[a]) for the crowd which had been with him for three days and refused to send them back to their homes without eating, for some of them had come a long distance (ἀπὸ μακρόθεν). Jesus is the only one in the narrative who noticed that they had nothing to eat. In this context, the verb of visual perception is implicit in the narrative. The heartfelt sensibility of the Lord for the crowd becomes explicit in his concern that some of them may collapse on the way back home. So in response to their physical need, Jesus proceeded to feed them (8:8), complementing the spiritual nourishment with the physical nutrition.

In both cases the narrative framework is optimistic and encouraging because the encounter initiated by Jesus' seeing has a positive outcome. The use of ἀπὸ μακρόθεν evokes an actual physical distance, whether it is the distance of the seeing, such as the demoniac's seeing in Mark 5:6[a], or the distance of the origin of the some of the followers of Jesus (Mark 8:3[b]), and connects it to the positive outcome in the narrative. In neither case is the distance depicted as an obstacle to being in a special relationship with the Lord. The apparent "long distance" in its physical dimension becomes a narrative device that highlights the power of the perception by a way of contrast.[2]

The text of Mark 15:40 establishes that some women (γυναῖκες) were observing (θεωροῦσαι) from a distance (ἀπὸ μακρόθεν). The allusion of the positive outcome evoked by the adverbial expression ἀπὸ μακρόθεν in Mark 5:6[a] and 8:3[b] seems to vanish in this context of the crucifixion of Jesus. But the positive outcome appears evident during the episode of the resurrection when the

---

1 Cf. Klemens Stock, *Boten aus dem Mit-Ihm Sein*: *Das Verhältnis zwischen Jesus und den Zwölf nach Markus* (AnBib 70; Roma: Pontificium Istitutum Biblicum, 1975), 7-70; Paul Danove, *The End of Mark's Story*: *A Methodological Study* (Leiden – New York – Köln: Brill, 1993), 258.

2 Cf. Paul Danove, "The Characterization and Narrative Function of the Women at the Tomb (Mark 15,40-41.47; 16,1-8)," *Bib* 77, no. 3 (1996): 379.

same women, who were observing from a distance, saw that the stone (θεωροῦσιν Mark 16:4[a]), which was very large, had been rolled away from the entrance of the sepulcher (Mark 16:1-4). The adverbial expression ἀπὸ μακρόθεν in the crucifixion narrative has been explained by Gnilka[3] and J. Marcus[4] as an allusion to Psalm 38:11: "Friends and companions stand aloof from my plague, even my kinsmen keep their distance (ἀπὸ μακρόθεν)." The distance of the women prevents their physical proximity with Jesus during his crucifixion, but it was not an obstruction for their love and faithfulness. According to the opinion of France, the distance (ἀπὸ μακρόθεν) in the narrative helps to create a contrast between the mocking onlookers and soldiers, who are close to the event of the cross, and the women, who despite being at a distance have an especial connection with the one who is crucified.[5]

The space between the observers and the object of their vision *per se* emphasizes the strength of the women's contemplation of the mystery in which they participate from a distance. Their watching implies a progression in time, so it was a constant prolonged action functioning as the permanent background of the scene. For this reason, it is described with θεωροῦσαι, the present active participle of the verb θεωρέω. Their observation is more than just a physical perception, because through their seeing (θεωροῦσαι) they participate in the mystery of the death of God's Son. Their speechless observation means that as perceivers, they are in a position of total reception toward the event of the crucifixion and its theological implications.

In the passage of Mark 15:41, the evangelist gives two qualitative notes about these women: a) they followed him when he was in Galilee (ἦν ἐν τῇ Γαλιλαίᾳ ἠκολούθουν αὐτῷ) and b) they were serving him (διηκόνουν αὐτῷ). The usage of the verb ἠκολούθουν evokes in the mind of the reader a narrative context of *sequela*, since the verb ἀκολουθέω,[6] "to follow," is used typically in Markan theology to indicate the basic action that characterized discipleship. The idea provokes a positive reaction in the reader's attitude towards the subject when Jesus is the object of the actions.[7] Subsequently, it is possible to conclude that Mark again provides the reader with the evocation of a narrative framework determined by the *sequela*, which can be illustrated with

3 Cf. Joachim Gnilka, *Das Evangelium nach Markus*. Evangelisch katolischer Kommentar zum NT (Zürich: Benziger Verlag 1979), II, 325.

4 Cf. Joel Marcus, *The way of the Lord: Christological Exegesis of the OT in the Gospel of Mark* (Edinburgh: T&T Clark, 1993), 174.

5 Cf. France, *The Gospel of Mark*, 663.

6 The verb ἠκολούθουν in Mark 15:41 is the indicative imperfect active 3rd person plural from ἀκολουθέω.

7 Cf. Mark 1:18; 2:14.15; 3:7; 5:24; 6:1; 8:34; 10:21.28.52; 11:9; 14:54.

the calling of the first disciples in Mark 1:16-29 and 2:14. In this manner, the evangelist evokes in the mind of his readers the narrative framework of discipleship as it is applied to the women (γυναῖκες) who, seen as disciples in this new narrative context of Jesus' death, present a clear contrast with the absence of the twelve during the passion and crucifixion.[8] "When all the male disciples have deserted, the women are still there, faithful to the last."[9] Furthermore, the faithful following of the women is complemented with a total spiritual observation of Jesus' death.

The same depiction of the women is maintained in Mark 15:47, where Mary Magdalene and Mary of Joses, without the explicit mention of Salome, continue observing where Jesus is laid: ἡ δὲ Μαρία ἡ Μαγδαληνὴ καὶ Μαρία ἡ Ἰωσῆτος ἐθεώρουν ποῦ τέθειται. This time their action is expressed in the imperfect tense, ἐθεώρουν, meaning that the action is sustained during the events of Jesus' crucifixion, death, and burial.[10] There is a dual purpose in their observation of the place of deposition of Jesus' body, τέθειται.[11] They were there not only simply to observe the place but also to know where to return after the Sabbath.

The narrative goes on in portraying the wordless women by placing their observation in the first narrative level with the verb in the indicative. The object of the main verb in the sentence is the body of Jesus and its place of burial, which functions as the point of reference for the encounter of the mystery of the empty tomb. The women's observation can be interpreted as a non verbal dialogue in the succession of these events.

On the first day of the week, Mary Magdalene, Mary the mother of James, and Salome, upon arriving to the tomb, looked up (ἀναβλέψασαι) and observed (θεωροῦσιν) that the stone had been rolled back (Mark 16:4). The action that the participle ἀναβλέψασαι describes is subordinate to the main verb in the sentence due to the sequence of tenses, because the central verb, θεωροῦσιν, is expressed in the present indicative. In its aorist active form, the participle ἀναβλέψασαι presents the action as simultaneously occurring with the principal verb in the narrative but at a secondary level. In addition to that important morphosyntactic feature, the "looking up" alludes to events where this participle precedes signifi-

---

8 Cf. Danove, "The Characterization," 379-380; France, *The Gospel of Mark*, 663; Raymond E. Brown, *The Death of the Messiah*: *From Gethsemane to the Grave. A Commentary on the Passion Narratives in the Four Gospels* (London: G. Chapman, 1994), 1155-1157.

9 France, *The Gospel of Mark*, 665.

10 Cf. Guerra-Gómez, *El idioma*, 303: Zerwick, *Biblical Greek*, n. 270-271.

11 Cf. France, *The Gospel of Mark*, 669. τέθειται is the indicative perfect passive 3rd person singular of the verb τίθημι.

cant actions of Jesus like the feeding of the crowd: καὶ λαβὼν τοὺς πέντε ἄρτους καὶ τοὺς δύο ἰχθύας *ἀναβλέψας* εἰς τὸν οὐρανὸν (6:41[a]), the healing of the deaf man: καὶ *ἀναβλέψας* εἰς τὸν οὐρανὸν ἐστέναξεν (7:34[a]), the healing of the blind man: καὶ *ἀναβλέψας* ἔλεγεν (8:24) and on other occasions with the connotation of regaining sight: ἵνα *ἀναβλέψω* / καὶ εὐθὺς *ἀνέβλεψεν* (10:51[b].52[b]). This action of "looking up" (ἀναβλέψας) is not enough for the evangelist, who wants to emphasize their perception with the verb θεωρέω that has as its direct object "the rolled stone" from the entrance of the empty tomb (ὅτι ἀποκεκύλισται ὁ λίθος Mark 16:4[a]). The γὰρ clause in 16:4[b] explains the great human obstacle that was resolved by a mysterious intervention: ἦν γὰρ μέγας σφόδρα .

The event of the open tomb exhibits similar characteristics to those presented in the context of the crucifixion and burial, namely:

a) The women's observation is not accompanied by any utterance.

b) The object of their observation continues to be the event of Christ's death that is not yet fully understood.

Their observation is not passive. In Mark 16:5, the author describes the next important action as the "entering" of the women into the tomb, for it is their distinctive watching that prompts them to go into the sepulcher: καὶ εἰσελθοῦσαι εἰς τὸ μνημεῖον εἶδον νεανίσκον. This time it is not just contemplation at a distance, but the perception of a mystery that invites them to enter into the inscrutability of the empty tomb, making the women instruments of the event of the risen Christ, so that they can continue to see and believe. Their entrance is complemented with the vision of the young man, (νεανίσκον) who, being a supernatural entity, announces the event of the resurrection (Mark 16:5-8). The young man appears sitting down. The description of the νεανίσκον with the present participle καθήμενον of the verb κάθημαι indicates the position of teaching, judgment,[12] and authority common in the Semitic culture.[13] The νεανίσκον is the person in the narrative who speaks with authority, proclaiming the good news of the resurrection from a location of burial. Through this detail, the author of Mark presents a paradox that can be explained from a theological point of view. The burial place, which signifies the reality of death and the summit of the power of

12 See Acts 23:3: "Then Paul said to him, 'God will strike you, you whitewashed wall. Do you indeed sit in judgment (κάθῃ κρίνων) upon me according to the law and yet in violation of the law order me to be struck?'" (NAB)

13 Cf. Moulton and Milligan, "κάθημαι," *VGNT*, 312.

men who condemned the Son of God, becomes the place of the authoritative announcement of life and the power of God that overcomes death itself.

The scene is very symbolic since the women came expecting a dead body, but ultimately they found an empty tomb where the only person inside is a young man dressed in white and seated in the place where Jesus was laid. The contrasts are sharp. Where the women expected the grief of a funeral, they found the young man who symbolizes the freshness of life. His white clothes also provides a contrast with the emotional state of the women and the atmosphere of the dark tomb.[14] The experience of the empty sepulcher becomes the first explicit sign of the accomplishment of the eschatological salvation that is not yet completely fulfilled in humanity.[15]

A reader can infer from these passages of Mark that the women's θεωρέω is not simply a physical observation of the events. In all three cases, the object of their perception is the reality of Jesus crucified (15:40-41), Jesus buried (15:47), and the open tomb (16:4), and so the object and the context determine the nature of their observation. In keeping with the line of thought from this contextual evidence and the theological key of the dialogues with Thomasios of John of Apamea, the reader can conclude that their physical perception implies a vision of faith that develops through the succession of the last dramatic episodes of Jesus' life. Subsequently, it is possible to conclude that the women's θεωρέω agrees with a physical observation, a *seeing* according to Wittgenstein's classification, that at the same time is able to go beyond the physical level to perceive a supernatural or divine dimension of Jesus' events. The *seeing as* of the women is characterized by the *intensity* of the event of Jesus' death and the empty tomb. The implications in their psyche touch the spiritual field, in which they become active participants and instruments of the divine economy of salvation.

14 Cf. France, *The Gospel of Mark*, 678-679.

15 Cf. Eugene Ruckstuhl, "Die evangelischen Ostererzählung," *Die Auferstehung Jesu Christi. Heilsgeschichtliche Tatsache und Brennpunkt des Glaubens*, eds. Eugene Ruckstuhl and Josef Pfammatter (Lucern: CiZ NF – München: Rex, 1968), 31-59. 53.

Conclusions

The episodes of visual perception treated above exhibit different semantic levels of comprehension that are connected to the aspect of seeing. The demons, for example, who are the characters in the narrative that function as the antagonists of the hero, portray a spiritual seeing capable of perceiving the divine manifestation hidden beneath the human condition, and as a result, they see Jesus as God (*seeing as*). In a similar way, Jesus sees with the eyes of God, catching sight of what is hidden to the human eye, but the effects of his seeing are radically opposed to the effects of the seeing of the demons. Therefore the spiritual seeing of these personages, Jesus and the demons, manifest diverse semantic levels that are incorporated in contexts of exorcisms, healing, divine manifestation of God, vocation, instruction, etc.

The women, on the other hand, represent an observation with faith by someone who keeps a spiritual and wordless dialogue from a distance, participating dynamically in the mystery of the death of Christ. The women see the crucifixion and burial of a loved one (*seeing*), but the divine nature of the event allows them to perceive the tragic event as a crucial moment of love and faith in the mystery of Jesus that is fully revealed and understood in the empty tomb (*seeing as*).

As a conclusion, I propose five lines of semantic dimension in which the action of the "spiritual seeing" is intrinsically related to different dimensions of understanding of the text.

1. The Seeing and the Christological Dimension

The passages explained in previous chapters manifest an essential relationship between "seeing" and Jesus' identity. In the beginning of Mark's Gospel, the double celestial object of Jesus' vision and the hearing of the divine voice of

God the Father establish the divine sonship of Jesus, a Trinitarian dimension that qualifies his Christological identity (Mark 1:10-11).[1] The encounters with the demoniacs continue along this same line of theological thought with the Christological confession manifested in the demons' voices as part of their characteristic reaction that always starts with a "seeing" and leads to the acknowledgement of the superior power of God. Their proclamation, which has its origin in their spiritual visual perception, expresses the truth about Jesus' personal identity. Their oral expression, however, is not equivalent to the divine voice of the Father in 1:11, because while the demoniacs react out of fear, expressing only the objective divine truth about the Son of God in Jesus, the utterance of the Father is expressed with a love that motivates the dynamic ministry of Jesus as a manifestation of the mission of the Logos, who progressively educates the disciples about his true identity as the Messiah.

Jesus' seeing of his disciples, the anonymous four men, the nameless woman with hemorrhages, and the poor widow, all indicate his awareness of his own identity as a master, teacher, healer, and forgiver of sins, which are fundamental characteristics of the divine and human nature that work conjunctly in his ministry. It is that consciousness which impels him to act accordingly, namely, as one who can call, heal, and restore the apparent distorted human condition, because he perceives the depth of the inner being of the ones who are called and healed.[2]

In this aspect, the contemplation of the women does not make the true identity of Christ as God explicit, but it does reveal the human nature of the one who truly died for the sake of love which is the essence of the Trinitarian God. The vision of the women demonstrates the reality of the death of the second person of the Trinity, and that implies an intense partaking of the mystery of God, who assumed the totality of the human nature.

2. The Seeing and a Dialogic Movement of Relationship

The dynamic expressed with the act of seeing can be described as a dialogue in which the one, who sees first, taking the initiative, provokes a reaction from the one who is seen. In this manner the interaction becomes dynamic, producing effective results that have a positive outcome, thanks to the presence of Jesus, who functions as the source of power and goodness.[3]

In the cases where the initiative belongs to Jesus, the reader recognizes that his seeing implies a personal connection with his interlocutors, provoking reac-

1 Cf. Palachuvattil, *"He saw,"* 263-264.

2 Cf. Palachuvattil, *"He saw,"* 262.

3 Cf. Boring, *Mark*, 274.

tions manifested in distinct forms of responses. In the particular episodes of vocation, the narrative reveals that the chosen ones acquire a special value and participation in the plot in the moment that they are "seen" by Jesus, almost as if they come into being in the moment that Jesus sees them. The divine initiative demonstrates that Jesus is always active, being the first to notice the presence of prospective disciples. The narration also indicates that in his seeing, Jesus is capable of catching a glimpse into the depth of the inner being of each person and in this way discovering the true aspects in each of them that are appreciated by God. For that reason, his "seeing" becomes the first step of a special rapport that is manifested explicitly through the calling to experience a *sequela Christi*. The vocation, therefore, is grounded in Jesus' seeing.[4] After the invitation to follow him, the disciples' response is active, radical, and silent. From that moment on, their relationship involves a continual growth in their personal knowledge of their master, which also implies a progressive conformation with the path of the Lord.[5] In the same way, Jesus' seeing is the stepping ground that establishes a relationship that can have an opposing outcome in a context of vocation, as it happens in the episode of the rich man, where his answer to the invitation of *sequela* turns out to be a silent and radical rejection of Jesus' invitation to follow him (Mark 10:17-22).

In the episodes of exorcism, the initiative for the seeing belongs to the demons, who are the first ones to recognize the divine presence of the Son of God in the human appearance of Jesus. The double inter-relational movement starts with the demons, who always provoke in Jesus a reaction that has its end in the complete healing and restoration of the possessed person. The dynamic of the encounter, narrated according to the human level, manifests the divine reality hidden in the human appearance. The episodes described in Mark 3:11-12; 5:6-7; and 9:20 manifest a clash between the two basic forces: good and evil, which at the same time transport the reader to an eschatological level that incarnates the eternal battle of the universal cosmic forces where always the power of God and of Jesus always prevails against the evil forces that pursue the destruction of harmony and balance in the human condition.[6]

The women represent the disciples who contemplate the mystery of Christ. At that time, everything that was visible to the eyes of the women was verifiable: they were *seeing* Jesus crucified. They participate in a silent and spiritual communication based upon the spiritual sense of sight by visually perceiving a veiled mystery. Thus the possibility of catching a glimpse of the divine enigmas

4 Cf. Palachuvattil, *"He saw,"* 264.267-268.

5 Cf. Suzanne Watts Henderson, *Christology and Discipleship in the Gospel of Mark* (Cambridge, UK: Cambridge University Press, 2006), 241-243.

6 Cf. France, *The Gospel of Mark*, 366-367.

is part of the innate essence of the human soul, which has the *capax* of knowing spiritually but always through a given grace.

Following the theological thought of John of Apamea, the spiritual experience of the women goes beyond the physical senses, perceiving the divine manifestation on the cross. Thus with the senses of the soul, the women can begin to comprehend the divine mysteries manifested in the present moment, which contains conjointly the inscrutability of the Trinitarian mysteries of love. Hence, it is possible to read and understand the episode of the crucifixion as a spiritual communication that is achievable because God can speak to a person without the physical sound of his voice, establishing a new dialogue in the invisible and spiritual intimacy between the spiritual senses of the women and himself.

3. The Seeing and the Healing Dimension of the Human Condition

The previous point leads us to the fact that Jesus' seeing initiates a chain reaction that is manifested in the unfolding of a series of events and concludes with the total renovation and healing of the possessed person. The demons destroy the harmonious balance of social living that the person had during the pre-possessed state, to the point of isolating him or her from other persons and even from God himself. Therefore the stories of exorcism bear implicitly a context of healing, since they describe the re-establishment of the ideal state of communication and functionality of the person within the social community and with the personal God of Jesus.

Other episodes of healing are characterized by the absence of demons. These episodes are the cases of the paralytic man in Mark 2:1-5 and the anonymous woman with hemorrhages in Mark 5:31-32. In both narratives, the process of healing begins with Jesus' seeing, which implies more than just a physical perception of the reality in front of him. In the first case, Jesus perceives the inner being of the four anonymous bearers of the paralytic, recognizing the faith grounded in their hearts. This turns out to be the basic condition that motivates the total healing of soul and body of the one who could not walk on his own to encounter the Lord. The other episode narrates the courage of a nameless woman who seeks her own physical renewal, but Jesus' seeing examines the complex reality of the ill person in order to provide an integral healing that establishes the ground for a new path of faith. When Jesus in Mark 5:34 declares to the unnamed woman that her faith has saved her, the evangelist used the verb σῴζω in perfect indicative active: σέσωκέν, in order to indicate a healing that goes beyond a simply physical healing, a cure that includes her body and soul, namely, a total renewal of her human condition. That outcome endures in time to the extent that the personal encounter with Jesus produces a permanent state of liberated life for the woman who was condemned and excluded from her society because of her physical condition.[7]

4. Jesus' Seeing and a Didactic Dimension

The pedagogical aspect of Jesus' seeing is manifested explicitly in the episode of the poor widow in Mark 12:41-44. The narrative does not describe a context of exorcism or healing; Jesus is simply observing "how" the people were putting their offering. His persistent and spiritual contemplation of the human condition motivates him to impart an instruction to his closest friends, the disciples (12:43[a]). The purpose of the didactic communication described in the direct style of discourse in 12:43[b]-44, is to educate the disciples *in seeing as God sees*, which means growing in the capacity to perceive the reality with the spiritual eyes in order to discover what is hidden to the human sight since man looks to the outward appearance of every situation but Jesus, whose seeing proves God's manner of seeing, perceives the soul and the heart. This attitude of Jesus echoes the instruction of Yhwh to Samuel when Samuel chooses David, for the Lord said to Samuel: "do not look (ἐπιβλέψης) at his appearance, or on the height of his stature, because I have rejected him; for God does not see (ὄψετα) as man sees (ἐμβλέψεται). For man looks (ὄψεται) at the outward appearance, but God looks at the heart (ὁ δὲ θεὸς ὄψεται εἰς καρδίαν)" (1Sam 16:7).

5. Pragmatic Dimension of the Texts

The pericopes studied using the notion of the spiritual senses as developed in the writings of John of Apamea, in addition to those of Origin, Bonaventure, and Ignatius of Loyola, lead us to read Mark's Gospel from a pragmatic perspective, which is an extension of the semantic analysis of the episodes. A pragmatic reading leads us to question the purpose of the text, namely, for what were these narrations written? What is the importance for the modern reader? What do the episodes ask the reader to do?[8]

The Gospel narratives were written to inform an audience—the real audience of the Gospel or seekers of God—about the truth of the event of Christ, so

7 Cf. Xabier Pikaza, *Para vivir el evangelio. Lectura de Marcos* (Estella, Navarra: Editorial Verbo Divino, 1995), 81.

8 Cf. Brigitte Schlieben-Lange, *Linguistische Pragmatik.* UTB 198 (Stuttgart: Kohlhammer, 1979), 97.

they have a fundamental informative dimension. The written kerygma is also intended to persuade the reader to believe in what is recounted and act upon that belief, having a practical aspect that motivates to act upon what is communicated. Therefore the content of these particular Gospel episodes must be considered in light of the end for which they were written, which is an active participation of the readers independently of the place and time in which are situated.[9]

At this point, the episodes that describe Jesus' seeing have a "directive function," which is also referred to as "conative," motivate the reader to act by way of imitation and identification with the character in the narration.[10] The pericopes present to the reader a pragmatic way to follow and to practice in his or her daily life the spiritual seeing that is portrayed in Jesus. Along this line of thought, the author of Mark makes this intention explicit with the didactic instruction of Jesus to his disciples regarding the situation of the poor widow (12:41-44). The author of Mark emphasizes how the seeing of Jesus portrays an educational moment for the disciples, so that they will learn how to perceive the human reality according to the mindset of God. In the same manner, the author wants to transmit this way of seeing to his community, into which every Christian community, that reads and meditates on the kerygmatic episodes noting visual perception, throughout the course of history is incorporated.

At this point, it is certainly useful to apply the criteria established by Origen and echoed in the thoughts of John of Apamea. Through the practice of the spiritual senses, especially the spiritual sense of sight, a person can experience the divine immersed and hidden in the human condition. This way of perception is, for the most part, unfruitful or absent in daily lives because the spiritual senses are dystrophic. This condition of abnormal development often denotes the degeneration in the spiritual life due to the lack of perception of God's action in the unfolding of the human events. For this reason, therapeutic exercise of the soul's senses is required in order to begin spiritual growth so that the spiritual senses will be awakened, since that is the first step of their development, being accomplished by their daily implementation. The Ignatian spiritual exercises, in this aspect, are an excellent way of awaking the senses of the soul that are numb due to their lack of use. Through the stirring of the soul's senses, it is possible for the reader-believer to develop his or her perception to the point that he or she is able to perceive the reality of God and the manifestation of evil through the outward appearance of human circumstances.

---

9 Cf. Wilhem Egger, *Methodenlehre zum Neuen Testament. Einführung in linguistische und historisch-kritische Methoden* (Freiburg – Basel –Wien: Herder, 1987), 133-135.

10 Cf. Rémi Lack, *Letture strutturaliste dell'Antico Testamento* (Roma: Edizione Borla, 1978), 25-28; Egger, *Methodenlehre zum Neuen Testament*, 140-142.

Bibliography

Abrahams, Israel. *Studies in Pharisaism and the Gospels*. New York, NY: Ktav Publishing House, 1967.

Asemani, Giusseppe Simone. *Bibliotheca Orientalis Clementino-Vaticana: In Qua Manuscriptos Codices Syriacos, Arabicos, Persicos, Turcicos, Hebraicos, Samaritanos, Armenicos, Aethiopicos, Graecos, Aegyptiacos, Ibericos, et Malabaricos, jussu et munificentia Clementis XI Pontificis Maximi ex Oriente Conquisitos, Comparatos, et Bibliotecae Vaticanae Addictos Recensuit, Digessit, et Genuina Scripta a Spuriis Secrevit, Addita Singulorum Auctorum Vita, Joseph Simonius Assemanus, Syrus Maronita*. Rome: Typis Sacrae Congregationis de Propaganda Fide, 1719–1728. I-IX. Reprint: Charleston, SC: Nabu Press, 2011.

Augustine of Hippo. "Sermons" (From the Gospel of Mark). In *PLS* 2:424–427; *PL* 38:581–591; 1104–1107; 1112–1115; 1126–1133.

———. "Sermons" (From the Gospel of Mark). In *NPNF* 1, 6:406–413, translated by R. G. MacMullen and edited by Philip Schaff.

———. "Sermons 94A–147A on the NT." In *The Works of Saint Augustine: A Translation for the 21st Century*, translated by Edmund Hill. Brooklyn, NY: New City Press, 1992.

Balás, David L., and Binham Jeffrey. "Patristic Exegesis of the Books of the Bible". In *Handbook of Patristic Exegesis*, edited by Charles Kannengiesser, 273-373. Leiden – Boston: Brill, 2004. I.

von Balthasar, Hans Urs. *The Glory of the Lord: A Theological Aesthetics. Seeing the Form*. San Francisco: Ignatius Press, 1982. I.

Barr, James. "Childs' Introduction to the Old Testament as Scripture," *JSOT* 16 (1980): 12-23.

Bauer, Walter A. *Greek-English Lexicon of the New Testament and Other Early Christian Literature*. Original title: *Grieschische-Deutsches Wörterbuch zu den Schriften des Neuen Testaments und der übrigen urscristlichen*

Literatur. Translated by William Arndt and Wilbur Gingrich. Chicago, IL: Chicago University Press, 1979.

Baumstark, Anton. *Geschichte der Syrischen Literatur*: *Mit Ausschluss der Christlich-Palästinensischen Texte*. Bonn: A. Markus und E. Webers Verlag, 1922.

Beardsley, Monroe. *Aesthetics: Problems in the Philosophy of Criticism*. New York: Harcourt, Brace, 1958.

Bedjan, Paul. *Homiliae S. Isaaci Syri Antiocheni*. Paris – Leipzig: Harrassowitz Verlag, 1903. I.

______. *Mar Isaacus Ninivita. De Perfectione Religiosa*. Paris – Leipzig: Harrassowitz Verlag, 1909.

Blass, Friederich Wilhem, and Debrunner Albert. *Grammatica del Greco del Nuevo Testamento*. Edited by Friederich Rehkopf. Brescia: Paideia, 1997.

Böhm, Thomas. "The Problem of Senses as Methods of Exegesis: Allegory and History." In *Handbook of Patristic Exegesis*, edited by Charles Kannengiesser, 212-228. Leiden – Boston: Brill, 2004. I.

Boring, Eugene. *Mark. A Commentary*. NTL. Louisville – London: Westminster John Knox Press, 2006.

Borrett, Marcel, ed. *Origen, Contre Celse*. SC 147. Paris: Les Éditions du Cerf, 1969.

Brock, Sebastian. *The Syriac Fathers on Prayer and the Spiritual Life*. Kalamazoo, MI: Cistercian Publications, 1987.

Brown, Raymond E. *The Death of the Messiah: From Gethsemane to the Grave. A Commentary on the Passion Narratives in the Four Gospels*. London: G. Chapman, 1994.

Büchsel, Friedrich. "ἀλληγορέω," *TDNT* I, 260-262.

Caner, Daniel. *Wandering, Begging Monks. Spiritual Authority and the Promotion of Monasticism in Late Antiquity*. Berkeley – Los Angeles – London, UK: University of California Press, 2002.

Childs, Brevard S. "The Canonical Shape of the Prophetic Literature," *Interpretation* 32 (1978): 46-55.

Clark, Walter H. "Seeing As and Knowing That in Aesthetic Education." In *Aesthetic Concepts and Education*, edited by Ralph A. Smith, 182-203. Urbana – Chicago – London: University of Illinois Press, 1970.

Clement of Alexandria. "Christ the Educator 1.4." In *Ante-Nicene Fathers*, edited by Alexander Roberts, James Donaldson, and Arthur C. Coxe. Peabody, MA: Hendrickson, 1994. II.

Corrigan, Kevin. *Evagrius and Gregory: Mind, Soul and Body in the 4th Century*. Ashgate Studies in Philosophy and Theology in Late Antiquity. Farnham, UK – Burlington, VT: Ashgate, 2009.

Cureton, William. *Corpus Ignatianum. A Complete Collection.* Berlin: Asher and Co., 1849.

Danove, Paul. "The Characterization and Narrative Function of the Women at the Tomb (Mark 15,40-41.47; 16,1-8)," *Bib* 77, no. 3 (1996): 375-397.

______. *The End of Mark's Story: A Methodological Study.* Leiden – New York – Köln: Brill, 1993.

Dedering Sven. ed. et trans. *Johannes von Lycopolis, Ein Dialog über die Seele und die Affekte des Menschen.* Leipzig – Uppsala – Haag: O. Harrassowitz Verlag, 1936.

Denzinger, Heinrich J. D. *Enchiridion Symbolorum, Definitionum et Declarationum de Rebus Fidei et Morum. The Sources of Catholic Dogma.* Translated by Roy J. Deferrari. St. Louis, MO – London, UK: Herder, 1957.

Donahue, John, and Harrington Daniel. *The Gospel of Mark.* Sacra Pagina 2. Collegeville, MN: The Liturgical Press, 2007.

Donaldson, James. "Called to Follow: A Twofold Experience of Discipleship in Mark," *BTB* 5 (1975): 67-77.

Dowd, Sharyn. *Reading Mark. A Literary and Theological Commentary on the Second Gospel.* Macon, GA: Smyth & Helwys, 2000.

Duchesne, Louis. *Early History of the Christian Church. From Its Foundation to the End of the Fifth Century.* London: John Murray Ltd., 1957. II.

Duval, Rubens. *La Littérature Syriaque.* Paris: V. Lacoffre, 1900.

Ebedjesu, Khayyath G. *Syri Orientales, seu Chaldaei, Nestoriani et Romanorum Pontificum Primatus. Commentatio Historico-Philologico-Theologica.* Syriac Studies Library 105. Piscataway, NJ: Gorgias Press 1870, 2011.

______. "Metrical Catalogue of Syriac Writers." In *The Nestorians and Their Rituals*, edited by G. P. Badger, 361-379. London: Joseph Masters and Co., 1852. II.

Edwards, James R. *The Gospel According to Mark.* Grand Rapids, MI: Eerdmans, 2002.

Ephrem the Syrian. "Commentary on Tatian's Diatessaron". Leloir 1990:88; JSSS 2:129. In *Mark. ACCS NT II*, edited by Thomas C. Oden and Christopher A. Hall. Downers Grove: InterVarsity Press, 2005.

Epiphanius of Salamis. *Panarion. Books II and II (Sects 47-80; De Fide).* Translated by F. Williams. Leiden – New York – Köln: Brill, 1993.

Egger, Wilhem. *Methodenlehre zum Neuen Testament. Einführung in Linguistische und Historisch-Kritische Methoden.* Freiburg – Basel –Wien: Herder, 1987.

Ettlinger, Gerard H. *Theodoret: Eranistes.* FC. Washington, DC: Catholic University of America Press, 2003.

Eusebius. "Historia Ecclesiastica 3.39.14–15". NPNF 2,1:172–173. In *Mark. ACCS NT II*, edited by Thomas C. Oden and Christopher A. Hall. Downers Grove: InterVarsity Press, 2005.

Flavius Josephus, "Jewish War 5.5.2." In *The Genuine Works of Flavius Josephus, the Jewish Historian*, translated by William Whiston. Boston 1737. accessed October 17, 2013. http: //www. ccel.org/ ccel/ josephus/ complete.iii.vi.v.html.

______. "Jewish War 6.5.2." In *The Genuine Works of Flavius Josephus, the Jewish Historian*, translated by William Whiston, accessed October 17, 2013. http://www.ccel.org/ccel/josephus/complete.iii.vii.v.html.

France, Richard Thomas. *The Gospel of Mark. A Commentary on the Greek Text*. NIGTC. Grand Rapids, MI – Cambridge, UK: Eerdmans and Paternoster Press Carlisle, 2002.

Freedman, Harry, and Maurice Simon, eds. *Midrash Rabbah, Genesis*. London, UK: Socino Press, 1961.

Foerster, Werner. "δαίμων," *TDNT* II, 1-20.

Frankenberg, Wilhem. *Evagrius Ponticus. Abhandlungen der Königlichen Gesellschaft der Wissenschaften zu Göttingen Philologisch-Historische Klasse.* Neue Folge 13, no. 2. Berlin: Weidmannsche Buchhandlung, 1912.

Gargano, Innocenzo. "La Metodologia Esegetica dei Padri." In *Metodologia dell'Antico Testamento*, edited by Horacio Simian-Yofre, 197-222. Bologna: Dehoniane, 1995.

______. *La Teoria di Gregorio di Nissa sul Cantico dei Cantici. Indagine su alcune indicazioni di metodo esegetico*. Roma: Pontificium Institutum Studiorum Orientalium, 1981.

Gnilka, Joachim. *Das Evangelium nach Markus*. Evangelisch Katolischer Kommentar zum Neuen Testament. Zürich: Benziger Verlag, 1979. II.

Gould, Ezra. *Critical and Exegetical Commentary on the Gospel According to St. Mark*. Edinburgh, UK: T&T Clark, 1961.

Greer, Rowan A. *Theodore of Mopsuestia. Exegete and Theologia*. London: Faith Press, 1961.

Grundmann, Walter. *Das Evangelium nach Markus*. THNT 2. Berlin: Evangelische Verlagsanstalt Berlin, 1977.

Gregory of Nyssa. *De Vita Moysis*. Edited by Herbert Musurillo. Leiden: Brill, 1964.

Griffith, Sidney H. "A Spiritual Father for the Whole Church: The Universal Appeal of St. Ephraem the Syrian," *Hugoye: Journal of Syriac Studies*, 1, no. 2 (1998): 197-220.

Guerra-Gómez, Manuel. *El idioma del Nuevo Testamento. Gramática, Estilística y Diccionario Estadístico del Griego Bíblico*. Facultad de Teología del Norte de España. Burgos: Ediciones Aldecoa, [4]1995.

Guillaumont, Antoine. *Les 'Kephalaia Gnostica' d'Evagre le Pontique et l'Histoire de l'Origénisme chez les Grecs et chez les Syriens*. Patristica Sorbonensia 5. Paris: Cerf, 1962.

Guillet, Jacques. "Les Exégèses d'Alexandrie et d'Antioche. Conflit ou Malentendu?," *RScR* 34 (1947): 257-302.

Guy, Jean-Claude. "Jean de Lycopolis," *DSAM* VI, 619-620.

Hadot, Pierre. *Philosophy as a Way of Life: Spiritual Exercises from Socrates to Foucault*. Oxford: Blackwell Publishing, 2003.

de Halleux, André. *Philoxène de Mabbog. Sa Vie, ses Écrits, sa Théologie*. Louvain: Impr. Orientaliste, 1963.

Harb, Paul. "Doctrine Spirituelle de Jean le Solitaire (Jean d'Apamée)," *PO 2* (1971): 225-260.

Harrington, Daniel J. "The Gospel According to Mark." In *The New Jerome Biblical Commentary*, edited by Raymond E. Brown, Joseph A. Fitzmyer, and Roland E. Murphy, 596-629. Englewood Cliffs, NJ: Prentice Hall, 1990.

Hausherr, Irenée, ed. et trans. *Jean le Solitaire (Pseudo-Jean de Lycopolis), Dialogue sur l'Âme et les Passions des Homes*. Traduit du Syriaque sur l'Edition de Sven Dedering. Orientalia Christiana Analecta 120. Roma: Pontificium Institutum Orientalium Studiorum, 1939.

______. "Un Grand Auteur Spirituel Retrouvé: Jean d'Apamée," *OCP* 14 (1948): 3-42.

Hay, Camillus. "The Christology of Theodore of Mopsuestia," *ABR* 9 (1961): 43-45.

Hendriksen, William. *The Gospel of Mark*. NTC. Grand Rapids, MI: Baker Book House, 1975.

Hengel, Martin. *The Charismatic Leader and His Followers*. Translated by James Greig. SNTW. Edinburgh: T&T Clark, 1996.

Hill, Robert C. "His Master's Voice: Theodore of Mopsuestia on the Psalms," *Heythrop Journal* 45, no. 1 (2004): 40-53.

Howard, Jackson M. "The Death of Jesus in Mark and the Miracle from the Cross," *NTS* 33 (1987): 16-37.

Hunt, Hannah. "The Tears of the Sinful Woman: A Theology of Redemption in the Homilies of St. Ephraim and his Followers," *Hugoye: Journal of Syriac Studies*, 1, no. 2 (1998): 165-184.

Ignatius of Loyola. *Spiritual Exercises*. Translated by Elder Mullan. New York: Kennedy and Sons, 1914.

van Iersel, Bas. *Mark. A Reader-Response Commentary*. London, UK – New York, NY: T&T Clark, 1998.

______, *Marco. La lettura e la Risposta. Un Commento*. Brescia: Queririana, 2000.

Jean le Solitaire (Pseudo-Jean de Lycopolis), *Dialogue sur l'Âme et les Passions des Homes*. Traduit du Syriaque sur l'Edition de Sven Dedering. Edited and translated by Irenée Hausherr. Orientalia Christiana Analecta 120. Roma: Pontificium Institutum Orientalium Studiorum, 1939.

Jean D'Apamée. *Dialogues et Traités*. Edited and translated by René Lavenant. SC 311. Paris: Les Éditions du Cerf, 1984.

Jerome (Pseudo-Chrysostom). *Tractatus 10 in Marci Evangelium*. Edited by D. G. Morin. Turnhout: Brepols, 1958.

———. CCSL 78:449–500.

———. "Homilies on the Gospel of Mark." In *The Homilies of St. Jerome*, translated by M. L. Ewald. Washington: Catholic University of America Press, 1964.

———. FC 57:121–192.

John Chrysostom. "Homily 12.3 of the Gospel of St. Matthew." In *NPNF* 1 10:77; *TLG* 2062.152,57.205.25-35, 41-47.

———. "Sermons" (From the Gospel of Mark). In *PG* 51:31–40; *PG* 58:603–610; 757–767.

Johannes von Apamea. *Drei Traktate von Johannes dem Einsiedler*. Edited and translated by Lars Gösta Rignell. Lund: C. W. K. Gleerup, 1960.

Johannes von Lycopolis. *Ein Dialog über die Seele und die Affekte des Menschen*. Edited and translated by Sven Dedering. Leipzig – Uppsala – Haag: O. Harrassowitz Verlag, 1936.

Juel, Donald. *A Master of Surprise: Mark Interpreted*. Minneapolis, MN: Fortress / Augsburg Fortress, 1994.

Kannengiesser, Charles. *Handbook of Patristic Exegesis*. Leiden – Boston: Brill, 2004. I.

Keck, Leander E. "Mark 3:7-12 and Mark's Christology," *JBL* 84 (1965): 341-358.

Kitchen, Robert A. *In Search of Lost Apophthemata in John the Solitary of Apamea*. Regina, Saskatchewan: Knox-Metropolitan United Church, Independent Academia, 2012.

Kovacs, Judith. "Human Participation in God's Plan: The Legacy of Clement of Alexandria," *JECS* 9, no. 1 (2001): 1-2.

______. "Divine Pedagogy and the Gnostic Teacher According to Clement of Alexandria," *JECS* 9, no. 1 (2001): 3-25.

Labourt, Jérôme. *Le Christianisme dans l'Empire Perse sous la Dynastie Sassanide*. Bibliotheque de l'Enseignement de l'Histoire Ecclesiastique. Paris: V. Lecoffre, ^{2}1904.

Lack, Rémi. *Letture Strutturaliste dell'Antico Testamento*. Roma: Edizioni Borla, 1978.

Lang, Friedrich G. "Sola Gratia im Markusevangelium: Die Soteriologie des Markus nach 9,14-29 und 10,17-31." In *Rechtfertigung: Festschrift für Ernst Käsemann zum 70 Geburtstag*, edited by Johannes Friedrich, Wolfgang Pöhlmann, and Peter Stuhlmacher, 321-337. Tübingen: J. C. B. Mohr Vandenhoeck und Ruprecht, 1976.

Lagrange, Marie-Joseph. *Évangile Selon St. Marc*. Paris: Librairie Lecoffre. J. Gabalda et Co Editeurs, 1966.

Lavenant, René, ed. *Jean D'Apamée. Dialogues et Traités*. Introduction, Traduction et Notes. SC 311. Paris: Les Éditions du Cerf, 1984.

______. "Le Problème de Jean d'Apamée," *OCP* 46 (1980): 367-390.

______. "La Lettre à Patricius d'Édesse de Philoxéne de Mabboug," *PO* 30, no. 5 (1963): 723-883.

Lebon, Joseph. *Le Monophysisme Sévérien*. Louvain: Imprimerie Orientaliste, 1909.

______. "La Christologie du Monophysisme Syrien." In *Das Konzil von Chalkedon. Geschichte und Gegenwart*, edited by Aloys Grillmeier and Heinrich Bacht, 425-580. Würzburg: Echter Verlag, ^{5}1979. I.

van Leijsen, L. "De Driedeling van Het Geestelijk Leven bij Johannes van Apamea. Kritische Kanttekeningen bij enige Gangbare Interpretaties," *JECS* 51, no. 3-4 (1999): 213-240.

Liddell, Henry George, and Scott Robert. *Greek-English Lexicon*. Oxford, UK: The Clarendon Press, 1958.

Lightfoot, Joseph Barber. *The Apostolic Fathers*. Hildesheim – Zürich – New York: Georg Olms 1890, 1973. II/1.

de Lubac, Henri. "Typologie et Allegorisme," *RScR* 34 (1947): 180–226.

Llorca, Bernardino, García-Villoslada Ricardo, and Laboa Juan María. *Historia de la Iglesia Católica*. Madrid: BAC, 1996. I.

Marcus, Joel. *Mark 1-8*. AncB 27A. New York, NY – London, UK: Doubleday, 2000.

______. *The Way of the Lord: Christological Exegesis of the OT in the Gospel of Mark*. Edinburgh: T&T Clark, 1993.

Mateos, Juan, and Camacho Fernando. *Il Vangelo di Marco. Analisi Linguistica e Commento Esegetico*. Assisi: Cittadella Editrice, 1997. I-II.

McLeod, Frederik G. "Theodore of Mopsuestia Revisited," *ThS* 61, no. 3 (2000): 447-480.

McGuckin, John Anthony, ed. *The Book of Mystical Chapters. Meditations on the Soul's Ascent from the Desert Fathers and Other Early Christian Contemplatives*. Boston, MA – London, UK: Shambhala, 2003.

McKenzie, John. "Temple." In *Dictionary of the Bible,* 872-878. New York: Macmillan, 1965.

Michaelis, Wilhem. "ὁράω," *TDNT* V, 340-342.

Michel, Otto. "οἰκονομίαν," *TDNT* V, 151-153.

Michelson, David. "Introduction to Hugoye 13: A Double Issue to Philoxenos of Mabbug," *Hugoye: Journal of Syriac Studies*, 13, no. 1 (2010): 3-8.

Miller, Patricia Cox. *Dreams in Late Antiquity: Studies in the Imagination of a Culture*. Princeton, NJ: Princeton University Press, 1994.

Mingana, Alphonse. *Sources Syriaques*. Leipzig: Harrassowitz Verlag, 1907. I-II.

Motyer, Stephen. "The Rending of the Veil; A Markan Pentecost?," *NTS* 33 (1987): 155-157.

Moulton, James, and Milligan George. *The Vocabulary of the Greek Testament Illustrated from the Papyri and Other Non-Literary Sources*. Grand Rapids, MI: Eerdmans, 1982.

Neirynck, Frans. "Synoptic Problem." In *The New Jerome Biblical Commentary*, edited by Raymond E. Brown, Joseph A. Fitzmyer, and Roland E. Murphy, 587-595. Englewood Cliffs, NJ: Prentice Hall, 1990.

Nestle–Aland, *Novum Testamentum Graece*. Berlin: Deutsche Bibelgesellschaft 28th edition, 2012.

Oden Thomas C., and Hall Christopher A. eds. *Mark. ACCS NT II.* Downers grove: InterVarsity Press, 2005.

Origen. *Homilies on Leviticus. The Fathers of the Church*. Translated by Gary W. Barkley. Washington: Catholic University Press, 1990.

_____. *Contra Celsum*. Translated by Henry Chadwick. Cambridge – New York: Cambridge University Press, 1980.

_____. *Commentary on the Gospel according to John*, Books 1-10. Translated by R. E. Heine. FC 80. Washington: Catholic University of America Press, 1989.

_____. *Homilies on Genesis and Exodus*. Translated by R. E. Heine. FC 71. Washington: Catholic University of America Press, 1982.

_____. *An Exhortation to Martyrdom; Prayer; First Principles. Book IV. Prologue to the Commentary on the Song of Songs; Homily XXVII on Numbers*. Translation and Introduction by Rowan Greer. Classics of Western Spirituality. New York: Paulist Press, 1979.

_____. *On First Principles*. Translated by G. W. Butterworth. Gloucester, MA: Peter Smith, 1973.

_____. *On John's Gospel*. Edited by A. E. Brooke. Cambridge, UK: Cambridge University Press, 1896. I-II.

Ort, Lodewijk Josephus Rudolf. *Mani: A Religio-Historical Description of His Personality*. Leiden: Brill, 1967.

Ortíz de Urbina, Ignacio. *Patrologia Syriaca*. Roma: Pontificium Institutum Orientalium Studiorum, 1965.

Oswalt, John N. "Canonical Criticism: A Review From A Conservative Viewpoint," *JETS* 30, no. 3 (1987): 317-325.

Palachuvattil, Joy. *"He Saw." The Significance of Jesus' Seeing Denoted by the Verb Eiden in the Gospel of Mark*. Roma: Editrice Pontificia Universitá Gregoriana, 2002.

Palmer, Andrew. "A Single Human being divided in himself: Ephraim the Syrian, The Man in the Middle," *Hugoye: Journal of Syriac Studies*, 1, no. 2 (1998): 119-163.

_____. "The Influence of Ephraim the Syrian," *Hugoye: Journal of Syriac Studies*, 2, no. 1 (1999): 83-109.

Pásztori-Kupán, István. *Theodoret of Cyrus. The Early Church Fathers*. London – New York: Routledge, 2006.

Percival, Henry R., ed. *Council of Ephesus*. In the *Nicene and Post-Nicene Fathers*, 2nd Series. Digitalized by Fordham University, *Mediaeval Sourcebook: Council of Ephesus 431*. New York, 1996. XIV.

Pesch, Rudolf. *Il Vangelo di Marco*: *Parte prima. Testo Greco e Traduzione ai Cappitoli 1,1 - 8,26*. Brescia, Italia: Paideia, 1980.

Peter Chrysologus. *Sermons* (From the Gospel of Mark). Edited by Alexandre Olivar. Turnhout: Brepols, 1975.

———. "Sermons" (From the Gospel of Mark). In *CCSL* 24:102–105; 122–127; 167–172; 182–190; 206–210; 269–273; 284–291. *CCSL* 24A: 505–509; 511–516; 617–619. *CCSL* 24B: 1040–1049; 1054–1058; 1060–1064; 1068–1072.

———. "Sermons" (From the Gospel of Mark). In *FC* 17:75–80; 133–137; 276–282.

———. *Sermons* (From the Gospel of Mark). Edited by Alexandre Olivar. Turnhout: Brepols, 1981.

———. *Sermons* (From the Gospel of Mark). Edited by Alexandre Olivar. Turnhout: Brepols, 1982.

———. *Sermons* (From the Gospel of Mark). Translated by G. E. Ganss, 3–287. Washington: Catholic University of America Press, 1953.

Petruccione, John F., and Hill Robert C. *Theodoret of Cyrus. The Questions on the Octateuch. Greek Text and English Translation*. Washington, DC: Catholic University of America Press, 2007.

Pikaza, Xabier. *Para Vivir el Evangelio. Lectura de Marcos*. Estella, Navarra: Editorial Verbo Divino, 1995.

Plato. *The Republic*. Edited and translated by Desmond Lee. New York: Penguin Classics, 2007.

Powell, Mark A. *What is Narrative Criticism?* Minneapolis: Fortress Press, 1990.

Pseudo-Jerome. *Expositio Evangelii Secundum Markum*. Edited by M. Cahill. Turnhout: Brepols, 1997.

———. *Evangelium Secundum Markum*. In *CCSL* 82.

———. *The First Commentary on Mark: An Annotated Translation*. Translated by M. Cahill. New York: Oxford University Press, 1998.

———. *Commentarius in Evangelium Secundum Marcum*. In *PL* 30:589–644.

Pseudo-Theophilus. *Allegoriae in Evangelium Secundum Marcum*. In *PLS* 3:1308–1312.

Rahner, Karl. "Le Début d'une Doctrine des Cinq Sens Spirituels chez Origène," *RAM* 13 (1932): 113-145.

Resseguie, James L. *Narrative Criticism of the New Testament. An Introduction*. Grand Rapids, MI: Baker Academic Press, 2005.

Rengstorf, Karl H. "μαθητής," *TDNT* IV, 446-447.

Rignell, Lars Gösta, ed. *Briefe von Johannes dem Einsiedler mit Kritischem Apparat, Einleitung und Übersetzung*. Lund: Håkan Ohlssons Boktryckeri, 1941.

_____. *Johannes von Apamea, Drei Traktate von Johannes dem Einsiedler*. Lund: C. W. K. Gleerup, 1960.

Rosales-Acosta, Dempsey. *La Victoria Sobre el Poder de la Muerte. Ensayo Semántico y Narrativo del Texto Griego de Marcos 9:30-32*. Series Investigación. Sevilla: Círculo Rojo, 2012.

Ruckstuhl, Eugene. "Die evangelischen Ostererzählung." In *Die Auferstehung Jesu Christi*. Heilsgeschichtliche Tatsache und Brennpunkt des Glaubens, edited by Eugene Ruckstuhl and Josef Pfammatter, 31-59. CiZ NF; Lucern – München: Rex, 1968.

Sailhamer, John H. *Introduction to Old Testament Theology: A Canonical Approach*. Grand Rapids, MI: Zondervan Publishing House, 1995.

Sallustius. *Concerning the Gods and the Universe:* περί θεῶν και Κόσμου. Edited and translated with prolegomena by Arthur Darby Nock. Cambridge, UK: Cambridge University Press, 1926.

Schnackenburg, Rudolf. *Vangelo Secondo Marco*. Roma: Città Nuova Editrice, 2002.

Schneiders, Sandra M. *The Revelatory Text. Interpreting the New Testament as Sacred Scripture*. San Franciso: Harper, 1991.

Schlieben-Lange, Brigitte. *Linguistische Prgamatik*. UTB 198. Stuttgart: Kohlhammer 1979.

Scippa, Vincenzo. "Stile e Spunti di Teologia in Mc 5,21-43," *Asprenas* 30 (1983): 222-234.

Simonetti, Manlio. *Biblical Interpretation in the Early Church. An Historical Introduction to Patristic Exegesis*. Translated by J. A. Hughes. Edinburgh – New York: T&T Clark, 1994.

______. *Lettera e/o Allegoria. Un Contributo alla Storia dell'Esegesi Patristica*. Roma: Pontificium Institutum Patristicum Augustinianum, 1985.

Sieben, Hermann Josef. *Kirchenväterhomilien zum Neuen Testament: Ein Repertorium der Textausgaben und Übersetzungen, mit Einem Anhang der Kirchenväterkommentare*. Instrumenta Patristica 22. Steenbrugis: Abbatia S. Petri, 1991.

Simian-Yofre, Horacio ed. *Metodologia dell'Antico Testamento*. Bologna: Dehoniane, 1995.

Stadler, Ingrid. "On Seeing As," *Philosophical Review* 67 (1958): 91-94

Sterling, Gregory E. "Jesus as Exorcist: An Analysis of Matthew 17:14-20; Mark 9:14-29; Luke 9:37-43a," *CBQ* 55 (1993): 467-493.

Streeter, Burnett Hillman. *The Four Gospels: A Study of Origins, Treating of the Manuscript Tradition, Sources, Authorship, and Dates*. London: Macmillan, 1924.

Strothmann, Werner, ed. et trans. *Johannes vom Apamea, Sechs Gespräche mit Thomasios, Der Briefewechsel zwischen Thomasios und Johannes und drei an Thomasios gerichtete Abhandlungen*. Patristische Texte und Studien 11. Berlin: Walter de Gruyter, 1972.

Stock, Klemens. *Marco. Commento Contestuale al Secondo Vangelo*. Roma: Edizioni ADP, 2003.

______. *Boten aus dem Mit-Ihm Sein: Das Verhältnis Zwischen Jesus und den Zwölf nach Markus*. AnBib 70. Roma: Pontificium Institutum Biblicum, 1975.

Théodore Bar Koni. *Liber Scholiorum*. CSCO 66. Paris – Louvain: Louvain Catholic University Press, 1912.

Theodore of Mopsuestia. *Fragmenta in Marcum*. PG 66:713–716.

Thomas Aquinas. *Summa Theologica*. New York – Boston: Bezinger Brothers, 1947.

Ulansey, David. "The Heavenly Veil Torn: Mark's Cosmic Inclusio," *Bib* 110, no. 1 (1991): 123-125.

Völkel, M. "Γαλιλαία," *DENT*, I, 700-703.

Wallace, Daniel. *Greek Grammar Beyond the Basis. An Exegetical Syntax of the New Testament*. Grand Rapids, MI: Zondervan Publishing House, 1996.

Witherington III, Ben. *The Gospel of Mark. A Socio-Rhetorical Commentary*. Grand Rapids, MI – Cambridge, UK: Eerdmans, 2001.

Wittgenstein, Ludwig. *Philosophical Investigations*. Translated by Gertrude Elizabeth M. Anscombe. New York: Macmillan, 1953.

Wright, William. *Catalogue of Syriac Manuscripts*. London: British Museum of Oriental Printed Books and Manuscripts, 1838,1870.

______. *The Homilies of Aphraates, the Persian Sage. The Syriac Text*. London: Williams and Norgate, 1869. I.

Zerwick, Maximilian, *Biblical Greek*. Roma: Pontificium Istitutum Biblicum, 2001.

Index of Authors

Index of Subjects

Studies in Biblical Literature

This series invites manuscripts from scholars in any area of biblical literature. Both established and innovative methodologies, covering general and particular areas in biblical study, are welcome. The series seeks to make available studies that will make a significant contribution to the ongoing biblical discourse. Scholars who have interests in gender and sociocultural hermeneutics are particularly encouraged to consider this series.

For further information about the series and for the submission of manuscripts, contact:

Peter Lang Publishing
Acquisitions Department
29 Broadway, 18th floor
New York, NY 10006

To order other books in this series, please contact our Customer Service Department:

(800) 770-LANG (within the U.S.)
(212) 647-7706 (outside the U.S.)
(212) 647-7707 FAX

or browse online by series at:

WWW.PETERLANG.COM